Soft Tissue Sarcomas

Guest Editor

JOHN M. KANE III, MD

SURGICAL ONCOLOGY
CLINICS OF NORTH AMERICA

www.surgonc.theclinics.com

Consulting Editor
NICHOLAS J. PETRELLI, MD

April 2012 • Volume 21 • Number 2

SAUNDERS an imprint of ELSEVIER, Inc.

W.B. SAUNDERS COMPANY
A Division of Elsevier Inc.

1600 John F. Kennedy Boulevard • Suite 1800 • Philadelphia, PA 19103-2899

http://www.theclinics.com

SURGICAL ONCOLOGY CLINICS OF NORTH AMERICA Volume 21, Number 2
April 2012 ISSN 1055-3207, ISBN-13: 978-1-4557-3941-7

Editor: Jessica McCool
Developmental Editor: Teia Stone

Surgical Oncology Clinics of North America (ISSN 1055-3207) is published quarterly by Elsevier Inc., 360 Park Avenue South, New York, NY 10010-1710. Months of publication are January, April, July, and October. Business and Editorial Offices: 1600 John F. Kennedy Blvd., Ste. 1800, Philadelphia, PA 19103-2899. Customer Service Office: 3251 Riverport Lane, Maryland Heights, MO 63043. Periodicals postage paid at New York, NY and additional mailing offices. Subscription prices are $263.00 per year (US individuals), $386.00 (US institutions) $130.00 (US student/resident), $302.00 (Canadian individuals), $480.00 (Canadian institutions), $186.00 (Canadian student/resident), $377.00 (foreign individuals), $480.00 (foreign institutions), and $186.00 (foreign student/resident). Foreign air speed delivery is included in all *Clinics* subscription prices. All prices are subject to change without notice. **POSTMASTER**: Send address changes to *Surgical Oncology Clinics of North America*, Elsevier Health Science Division, Subscription Customer Service, 3251 Riverport Lane, Maryland Heights, MO 63043. **Customer Service: 1-800-654-2452 (US and Canada). 314-447-8871 (outside U.S. and Canada). Fax: 314-447-8029.** E-mail: journalscustomerservice-usa@elsevier.com (for print support); **journalsonline support-usa@elsevier.com** (for online support).

Reprints. For copies of 100 or more, of articles in this publication, please contact the Commercial Reprints Department, Elsevier Inc., 360 Park Avenue South, New York, New York 10010-1710. Tel. 212-633-3813; Fax: 212-462-1935; E-mail: reprints@elsevier.com.

Surgical Oncology Clinics of North America is covered in *MEDLINE/PubMed (Index Medicus)* and *EMBASE/ Excerpta Medica, Current Contents/Clinical Medicine,* and *ISI/BIOMED.*

Printed and bound by CPI Group (UK) Ltd, Croydon, CR0 4YY

Transferred to Digital Print 2012

Contributors

CONSULTING EDITOR

NICHOLAS J. PETRELLI, MD, FACS
Bank of America Endowed Medical Director, Helen F. Graham Cancer Center at Christiana Care Health System, Newark, Delaware; Professor of Surgery, Thomas Jefferson University, Philadelphia, Pennsylvania

GUEST EDITOR

JOHN M. KANE III, MD
Chief, Melanoma Sarcoma Service, Associate Professor, Department of Surgical Oncology, Roswell Park Cancer Institute, Buffalo, New York

AUTHORS

ZUBIN M. BAMBOAT, MD
Department of Surgery, Memorial Sloan-Kettering Cancer Center, New York, New York

CHARLES N. CATTON, MD, FRCP
Professor, Department of Radiation Oncology, University of Toronto; Radiation Medicine Program, Princess Margaret Hospital, Toronto, Ontario, Canada

THOMAS F. DELANEY, MD
Professor of Radiation Oncology, Harvard Medical School; Radiation Oncologist, Department of Radiation Oncology; Medical Director, Francis H. Burr Proton Therapy Center; Co-Director, Center for Sarcoma and Connective Tissue Oncology, Massachusetts General Hospital, Boston, Massachusetts

RONALD P. DEMATTEO, MD, FACS
Department of Surgery, Memorial Sloan-Kettering Cancer Center, New York, New York

TODD L. DEMMY, MD
Department of Thoracic Surgery, Roswell Park Cancer Institute; Department of Surgery, State University of New York-Buffalo, Buffalo, New York

JEREMIAH L. DENEVE, DO
Cutaneous Oncology Department, Moffitt Cancer Center, Tampa, Florida

MARCO L. FERRONE, MD
Department of Orthopedics, Brigham and Women's Hospital; Center for Sarcoma and Bone Oncology, Dana-Farber Cancer Institute; Instructor of Surgery, Harvard Medical School, Boston, Massachusetts

VALERIE FRANCESCUTTI, MD
Department of Surgical Oncology, Roswell Park Cancer Institute, Buffalo, New York

MELISSA E. HOGG, MD
Surgical Oncology Fellow, Department of Surgical Oncology, University of Pittsburgh Medical Center, Pittsburgh, Pennsylvania

HANS IWENOFU, MD
Assistant Professor, Department of Pathology, The Ohio State University, Columbus, Ohio

NATALIE B. JONES, MD
Clinical Instructor, Surgical Oncology Fellow, Department of Surgery, The Ohio State University, Columbus, Ohio

JOHN M. KANE III, MD
Chief, Melanoma Sarcoma Service, Associate Professor, Department of Surgical Oncology, Roswell Park Cancer Institute, Buffalo, New York

WILLIAM KRAYBILL, MD
Professor, Department of Surgery, The Ohio State University, Columbus, Ohio

STEVEN J. NURKIN, MD
Surgical Oncology, Roswell Park Cancer Institute, Buffalo, New York

SHREYASKUMAR PATEL, MD
Professor, Department of Sarcoma Medical Oncology, Houston, Texas

CHANDRAJIT P. RAUT, MD, MSc
Department of Surgery, Brigham and Women's Hospital; Center for Sarcoma and Bone Oncology, Dana-Farber Cancer Institute; Assistant Professor of Surgery, Harvard Medical School, Boston, Massachusetts

VINOD RAVI, MD
Assistant Professor, Department of Sarcoma Medical Oncology, Houston, Texas

THOMAS SCHARSCHMIDT, MD
Assistant Professor, Department of Orthopaedics, The Ohio State University, Columbus, Ohio

JOSEPH J. SKITZKI, MD
Assistant Professor, Departments of Surgical Oncology and Immunology, Roswell Park Cancer Institute, Buffalo, New York

RICHARD SMITH, MD
Department of Surgery, Tripler Army Medical Center; Department of Surgery, Cancer Research Center of Hawaii, Honolulu, Hawaii

CAROL J. SWALLOW, MD, PhD, FRCS, FACS
Professor, Department of Surgery and Institute of Medical Science, University of Toronto; Head, Division of General Surgery, Toronto Department of Surgical Oncology, Mount Sinai Hospital, Princess Margaret and Mount Sinai Hospitals, Toronto, Ontario, Canada

JEFFREY D. WAYNE, MD, FACS
Associate Professor of Surgery, Chief, Melanoma and Soft Tissue Surgical Oncology, Division of Gastrointestinal and Oncologic Surgery, Department of Surgical Oncology, Northwestern University Feinberg School of Medicine, Chicago, Illinois

JONATHAN S. ZAGER, MD, FACS
Associate Professor of Surgery, Cutaneous Oncology Department, Moffitt Cancer Center; Departments of Oncologic Sciences and Surgery, University of South Florida, Tampa, Florida

Contents

> Soft tissue sarcoma (STS) staging is a constantly evolving process. Grading is still of utmost importance and has been adapted into a three-tier system. The STS most difficult to categorize are those with uncertain malignant potential, such as solitary fibrous tumors, gastrointestinal stromal tumors, and glomus tumors, some of which have developed completely separate staging systems and may not even be considered sarcomas. Beyond the current TNM staging system, a multitude of prognostic factors for STS will continue to be discovered and ultimately incorporated into future revisions of the staging system.

> Historically the surgical management of extremity soft-tissue sarcomas (ESTS) commonly involved amputation. Nowadays limb-sparing, function-preserving surgery is the standard of care for ESTS. Adjuvant therapies such as radiation therapy and chemotherapy are used selectively in an effort to minimize both local recurrence and distant spread. Less common modalities, such as isolated limb perfusion, isolated limb infusion, and hyperthermia are being evaluated to potentially expand the cohort of individuals who may be eligible for limb-sparing surgery and to improve outcomes. This article reviews the standard and evolving approaches to the management of ESTS.

> Clinical trial data show that radiation enhances local tumor control of extremity sarcomas with acceptable morbidity when sophisticated radiation techniques are combined with limb-sparing resections performed by oncologic surgeons with sarcoma expertise. Similar controlled data is not available for retroperitoneal sarcomas but some studies suggest a benefit for radiotherapy. Radiation can be delivered by external beam or brachytherapy; it can be given pre-operatively, post-operatively, or intra-operatively. Indications for and advances in radiation therapy are discussed in this article.

Soft tissue sarcomas are rare mesenchymal neoplasms with considerable heterogeneity in biologic behavior and response to systemic therapy. Most patients present with localized disease and are potentially curable with multidisciplinary treatment. In patients with a high risk of developing metastatic disease, optimal use of neoadjuvant/adjuvant therapy has a definite role in improving patient outcomes by decreasing local and distant recurrences. Histology-specific clinical trials enrolling a homogenous high-risk population have been more successful in demonstrating benefit than larger trials with unselected heterogeneous patient populations. In specific histologic subtypes responsive to chemotherapy, neoadjuvant chemotherapy with close monitoring of response is recommended.

The relationship between surgical margin status and outcomes in sarcoma has been an area of controversy for years. Some question whether a positive margin represents inadequate surgery or perhaps is a marker of aggressive cancer biology. This article reviews the literature regarding the natural history of positive margins and its possible influence on sarcoma recurrence and survival.

The American Cancer Society predicts 10,520 new cases and 3920 deaths from soft tissue sarcoma (STS) for 2010. STS disseminates primarily via the hematogenous route, although lymphatic spread does occur with certain subtypes. The lung is the most common metastatic site in most large series, accounting for up to 80% of metastases. The median overall survival for pulmonary metastatic disease with current multidisciplinary treatment is approximately 12 to 14 months. Pulmonary metastasectomy (PM) represents the only potentially curative treatment for patients with STS and lung metastases. This article discusses the management of STS using PM.

Patients presenting with unresectable, large, primary or recurrent extremity soft tissue sarcoma or locally advanced extremity tumors may benefit from treatment options in the form of isolated regional perfusion therapy. Hyperthermic isolated limb perfusion (HILP) and isolated limb infusion (ILI) have proved to be efficacious with acceptable systemic and regional toxicity profiles. Both procedures are attractive as options for patients who might otherwise be facing amputation as limb salvage procedures. HILP and ILI can be offered as either definitive treatment or as neoadjuvant therapy followed by surgery and/or radiation treatment. Response rates are encouraging as are limb preservation rates after regional therapy. Ongoing multicenter collaborations and clinical trials are required to gain knowledge

evidence for an immunologic approach to sarcoma treatment. Initial clinical trials involving vaccines and adoptive immunotherapy have demonstrated promising results. The continued search for sarcoma tumor-associated antigens as specific targets is central to the clinical translation of effective immunotherapies.

VISIT THE CLINICS ONLINE!

Access your subscription at:
www.theclinics.com

Foreword

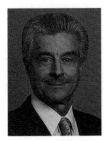

Nicholas J. Petrelli, MD
Consulting Editor

This issue of the *Surgical Oncology Clinics of North America* discusses sarcomas. The guest editor is John M. Kane III, MD, a surgical oncologist from the Roswell Park Cancer Institute in Buffalo, New York. Although sarcomas are rare tumors that account for less than 1% of all adult cancers, it does not supplant the fact that patients need to be treated at centers that have developed a multidisciplinary team approach to cancer care inclusive of extensive knowledge of the natural history of these tumors. Dr Kane has gathered together a group of experts who work in multidisciplinary teams to make sure patients receive proper and safe cancer care. The knowledge base needed to treat sarcomas starts with prognostic factors and understanding the staging for these tumors. William Kraybill, MD from The Ohio State University has spent his career treating patients with sarcomas and is an expert in this area. His article in this issue of the *Surgical Oncology Clinics of North America* is outstanding. Dr Kane, the guest editor, discusses margin status and its implications for local recurrence in this disease site. This article is a "must read" for physicians who care for these patients. Other articles, such as pulmonary metastasectomy by Todd Demmy, MD from Roswell Park and approaches to retroperitoneal sarcomas by Carol Swallow, MD from Mount Sinai Hospital in Toronto, discuss important treatment aspects of sarcomas with up-to-date information from the literature and their own experiences.

Gastrointestinal stromal tumors are rare tumors of the gastrointestinal tract. These tumors start in special cells found in the wall of the gastrointestinal tract called the interstitial cells of Cajal. These interstitial cells are part of the nervous system that regulates body processes, such as digesting food. The interstitial cells of Cajal have been labeled as pacemakers of the gastrointestinal tract because they send signals to the muscles in the digestive system allowing them to contract to move food and liquid through the gastrointestinal tract. Ron DeMatteo, MD from Memorial Sloan-Kettering Cancer Center has led the way in the management of gastrointestinal stromal tumors. He has written an outstanding article in the management of these tumors.

I would like to thank Dr John Kane and all of his colleagues for an outstanding issue of the *Surgical Oncology Clinics of North America*. Sarcomas need to be treated in

Surg Oncol Clin N Am 21 (2012) xiii–xiv
doi:10.1016/j.soc.2011.12.008
1055-3207/12/$ – see front matter © 2012 Elsevier Inc. All rights reserved.

surgonc.theclinics.com

experienced cancer centers where the multidisciplinary team of surgical, medical, and radiation oncologists formulates a plan of treatment. The authors in this issue of the *Surgical Oncology Clinics of North America* have demonstrated their expertise, and I thank them for their effort.

Nicholas J. Petrelli, MD
Helen F. Graham Cancer Center
4701 Ogletown-Stanton Road, Suite 1213
Newark, DE 19713, USA

E-mail address:
npetrelli@christianacare.org

Preface

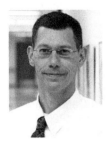

John M. Kane III, MD
Guest Editor

They Certainly Give Very Strange Names to Diseases
—Plato

Soft tissue sarcoma (STS) is a strange disease, indeed. Sarcoma comes from the Greek "sarx," meaning "flesh," and dates back to ancient times. It was not until the 1800s that STS was better understood as a cancer arising from embryonic mesoderm. STS accounts for approximately 1% of all adult cancers and the incidence has not really changed over time. It is this rarity that has both intrigued and challenged physicians caring for this disease.

What do we know and not know about STS? First, there are at least 40 different histologic subtypes. However, given our limited knowledge on the subject, most STS are clinically treated as one disease. Unfortunately, many of the nuances of biologic behavior are lost with this approach. Second, surgical resection with negative margins is the potentially curative treatment. However, the fact that STS can arise from any anatomic location means that the tumor is often in close proximity to critical structures. This frequently limits the ability to achieve widely negative margins without significant morbidity. In certain circumstances, radiation therapy can make up for not having a negative margin resection. However, when should radiation be considered versus when is surgery alone appropriate? Finally, despite the fact that local control is achieved in most extremity STS patients, 10%–50% will eventually succumb to distant metastatic disease. Clearly there must be a role for systemic therapies. Who? What? How long?

Unlike most other cancers, the scarcity of STS means that there will never be a significant number of large randomized trials to answer most of these important questions. The investigators worldwide who have completed the few prospective clinical trials for this disease should be applauded for their tenacity. It is only this limited scientific information as well as retrospective observations that we have at our disposal to make STS patient care decisions. Hopefully, this issue of *Surgical Oncology Clinics of North America* will provide a framework of knowledge to aid the clinician treating patients with this interesting and complex disease. Each article focuses on a topic that can sometimes vex the best of us. A few of the articles also highlight some successes and hope for the future of STS care.

Surg Oncol Clin N Am 21 (2012) xv–xvi
doi:10.1016/j.soc.2012.01.001
1055-3207/12/$ – see front matter © 2012 Elsevier Inc. All rights reserved.

surgonc.theclinics.com

I would like to thank the authors for their time and effort in creating this body of work. Without them, there would be no issue. I would also like to express sincere gratitude to my lead editor, Jessica McCool. Dealing with surgeons is always trying, especially with their "just-in-time" philosophy for project completion.

John M. Kane III, MD
Melanoma Sarcoma Service
Department of Surgical Oncology
Roswell Park Cancer Institute
Elm and Carlton Streets
Buffalo, NY 14263, USA

E-mail address:
John.Kane@RoswellPark.org

Prognostic Factors and Staging for Soft Tissue Sarcomas: An Update

Natalie B. Jones, MD[a], Hans Iwenofu, MD[b],
Thomas Scharschmidt, MD[c], William Kraybill, MD[a],*

KEYWORDS

• Soft tissue sarcoma • Staging systems • Genomic markers

INCIDENCE AND EPIDEMIOLOGY

Soft tissue sarcomas (STSs) represent fewer than 1% of all adult solid malignancies. In 2010, an estimated 10,520 new cases of STS and 3920 deaths occurred from the disease.[1,2] Overall 5-year survival for extremity STS is 50% to 90%; however, this varies greatly based on the grade and anatomic site. In general, the estimated 5-year survival is 25% to 50% for retroperitoneal sarcoma, which is poor compared with extremity STS. The prognosis for patients with high-grade retroperitoneal sarcoma is less favorable than for those with tumors at other sites because of the technical complexity of completely resecting these tumors and limitations to delivering high-dose radiation therapy to the abdomen.[3–6] The foundation for staging and grading systems for STS arose in the late 1970s and early 1980s when a task force convened to discuss these issues[7] after one of the earliest publications on staging.[8]

STSs are putatively derived from the mesenchymal cells during embryologic development, including fibrous connective tissue, fat, smooth or striated muscle, vascular tissue, peripheral neural tissue, and visceral tissue. Approximately 50% to two-thirds involve the extremities and 40% the trunk and retroperitoneum, with approximately 10% arising from the head and neck.[9] The most common subtypes are malignant fibrous histiocytoma (pleomorphic undifferentiated sarcoma), liposarcoma, leiomyosarcoma, synovial sarcoma, and malignant peripheral nerve sheath tumor (**Table 1**).[10] In children, rhabdomyosarcoma is the most common STS, although it ranks as seventh

[a] Department of Surgery, The Ohio State University, 410 West 10th Avenue, N924 Doan Hall, Columbus, OH 43210, USA
[b] Department of Pathology, The Ohio State University, 410 West 10th Avenue, N924 Doan Hall, Columbus, OH 43210, USA
[c] Department of Orthopedics, The Ohio State University, 410 West 10th Avenue, N924 Doan Hall, Columbus, OH 43210, USA
* Corresponding author.
E-mail address: william.kraybill@osumc.edu

Surg Oncol Clin N Am 21 (2012) 187–200
doi:10.1016/j.soc.2011.12.003
1055-3207/12/$ – see front matter © 2012 Elsevier Inc. All rights reserved.

Table 1
Histologic subtypes of soft tissue sarcomas

Histologic Subtypes	n	%
Malignant fibrous histiocytoma	349	28
Liposarcoma	188	15
Leiomyosarcoma	148	12
Synovial sarcoma	125	10
Malignant peripheral nerve sheath tumor	72	6
Rhabdomyosarcoma	60	5
Fibrosarcoma	38	3
Ewing's sarcoma	25	2
Angiosarcoma	25	2
Osteosarcoma	14	1
Epithelioid sarcoma	14	1
Chondrosarcoma	13	1
Clear cell sarcoma	12	1
Alveolar soft part sarcoma	7	1
Malignant hemangiopericytoma	5	0.4

Modified from Cormier JM, Pollock RE. Soft tissue sarcomas. CA Cancer J Clin 2004;54:94–109.

overall when combining adults and children. Other entities not included are Kaposi sarcoma, malignant extrarenal rhabdoid tumor, malignant tenosynovial giant cell tumor, malignant ossifying fibromyxoid tumor, malignant perivascular epithelioid cell tumors, desmoplastic round cell tumor, malignant glomus tumor, malignant triton tumor, and malignant gastrointestinal stromal tumor. Terminology for two of the listed tumors in **Table 1** has been altered to *malignant hemangiopericytoma-solitary fibrous tumor* and *Ewing's sarcoma/primitive neuroectodermal tumor*. With ongoing improvements in molecular pathology, probably more than 50 histologic subtypes of STS exist.

Despite the variety of histologic subtypes, STSs have many clinical and pathologic features in common. Because STSs are biologically similar and traditionally treated the same, this allows for common staging systems, which may not be appropriate. The American Joint Committee on Cancer (AJCC) staging system attempts to incorporate this commonality through only addressing anatomic depth, grade, and size of the tumor.

STSs metastasize primarily via a hematogenous route, particularly to the lungs. Lymph node metastasis is rare (<5%), except for a few histologic subtypes, such as epithelioid sarcoma, synovial sarcoma, rhabdomyosarcoma, clear-cell sarcoma, and angiosarcoma.[11] Local control is the primary treatment goal, with acceptable limb salvage rates for extremity STS. Selective metastasectomy also has a role. Five-year overall survival for patients who undergo metastasectomy is 30% if all metastatic disease is resected.[12]

Although the development of most STS is spontaneous, some STSs occur after a previous insult or exposure to carcinogenic agents. Radiation exposure accounts for only approximately 5% of all STSs, but a history of external beam radiation (e.g., for breast, cervix, ovarian, or lymphatic malignancies) is a well-known risk factor with an 8- to 50-fold increased incidence.[13,14] The risk of STS is directly related to the dose of radiation, and there appears to be a latency period of approximately 10 years. The most common histologic subtypes of radiation-associated sarcoma are extraskeletal osteogenic (21%), malignant fibrous histiocytoma (16%), and angiosarcoma/lymphangiosarcoma (15%). Most of these tumors (87%) are also high grade. Other risk factors include exposure to certain chemicals, including herbicides such as phenoxyacetic acids, and wood preservatives such as chlorophenols.[15,16] Chronic lymphedema after axillary node dissection has been associated with lymphangiosarcoma, otherwise known as Stewart-Treves syndrome.[17] Lymphangiosarcoma has also been associated with filarial infections and congenital lymphedema, seen predominantly on the lower extremities.[18] Certain viruses are linked to the development of sarcomas, including human immunodeficiency virus 1, human herpes virus 8 in Kaposi's sarcoma, and Epstein-Barr Virus in leiomyosarcoma.

GENETICS

Genetic mutations in mesenchymal stem cells give rise to malignant clones. STS are sometimes associated with specific inherited genetic alterations, but most have complex karyotypes. Numerous oncogenes have been implicated in the development of STS, including MDM2 (liposarcoma), N-myc (Ewing sarcoma), c-erbB2 (Ewing sarcoma), and members of the ras family (malignant fibrous histiocytoma, embryonal rhabdomyosarcoma). In addition to being important for diagnostic purposes, amplification of several of these genes in specific STS subtypes has been associated with a worse outcome.[19] Mutations in specific oncogenes result in chromosomal translocations that are associated with some histologic subtypes of STS. For instance, Ewing's sarcoma is associated with EWS-FLI1 fusion, clear cell sarcoma with EWS-ATF1 fusion, myxoid liposarcoma with TLS-CHOP fusion, alveolar rhabdomyosarcoma with PAX3-FHKR fusion, desmoplastic small round-cell tumor with EWS-WT1 fusion, and synovial sarcoma with SSX-SYT fusion (**Table 2**).[20,21] All of these tumors are

Table 2
Fusion genes in sarcomas

Sarcoma Type	Chromosomal Translocation	Fusion Gene	Year Reported
Ewing sarcoma	t(11;22)(q24;q12)	EWS-FLI1	1992
	t(21;22)(q22;q12)	EWS-ERG	1993
Clear cell sarcoma	t(12;22)(q13;q12)	EWS-ATF1	1993
Desmoplastic small round cell tumor	t(11;22)(p13;112)	EWS-WT1	1994
Extraskeletal myxoid chondrosarcoma	t(9;22)(q22;q12)	EWS-CHN	1995
Myxoid/round cell liposarcoma	t(12;16)(q13;p11)	TLS-CHOP	1993
Angiomatoid fibrous histiocytoma	t(12;16)(q13;p11)	TLS-ATF1	2000
Alveolar rhabdomyosarcoma	t(2;13)(q35;q14)	PAX3-FKHR	1993
	t(1;13)(p36;q14)	PAX7-FKHR	1994
Extraskeletal myxoid chondrosarcoma	t(9;17)(q22;q11)	TAF2N-CHN	1999
Synovial sarcoma	t(X;18)(p11;q11)	SYT-SSX1,2	1994
Dermatofibrosarcoma protuberans	t(17;22)(q22;q13)	COL1A1-PDGFB	1997
Congenital fibrosarcoma	t(12;15)(p13;q25)	ETV6-NTRK3	1998
Inflammatory myofibroblastic tumor	t(2p23)	Various ALK fusions	2000
Alveolar soft part sarcoma	t(X;17)(p11;q25)	ASPL-TFE3	2001
Endometrial stromal sarcoma	t(7;17)(p15;q21)	JAZF1-JJAZ1	2001

Modified from Borden EC, Baker LH, Bell RS, et al. Soft tissue sarcomas of adults: state of the translational science. Clin Cancer Res 2003;9:1941–56.

considered high-grade STSs and are most often associated with extensive cytogenetic abnormalities. Multiple inherited syndromes have STS components, including neurofibromatosis type I, retinoblastoma, Li-Fraumeni syndrome, Gardner syndrome, Werner syndrome, Gorlin syndrome, Carney triad, and tuberous sclerosis.[12]

In addition to oncogenes, tumor suppressor genes can be inactivated by either hereditary or sporadic mechanisms, and allow for uninhibited growth of tumor cells. Two tumor suppressor genes that are particularly relevant to STS are retinoblastoma (Rb-1) and p53. Mutations or deletions in the Rb gene can result in the development of retinoblastomas and sarcomas of soft tissues and bone. Mutations in the p53 tumor suppressor gene are the most common cytogenetic alteration in all human solid tumors, and have been associated with 30% to 60% of all STS.[22,23] Li-Fraumeni syndrome is also associated with this mutation.

CLINICAL PRESENTATION AND STAGING

The most common clinical presentation of STS is a painless and gradually enlarging mass. Sometimes trauma to the site may call attention to the presence of the sarcoma, but trauma is not necessarily a causative factor. In general, tumors of the thigh and retroperitoneum are larger on initial presentation than distal extremity tumors, because these spaces can conceal a mass much longer before it becomes noticeable. Often a zone of compression or pseudocapsule exists if no anatomic constraints are present, which can lead to pressure, paresthesias, distal edema, or bowel obstruction. Pseudocapsules will almost always have viable tumor in them, particularly in high-grade tumors. Different histologies can have varying growth rates and associated effects on the surrounding normal tissues. For example, liposarcoma is characteristically a "pushing" tumor, whereas synovial sarcoma is infiltrative.

Preoperative imaging is essential for surgical planning (for the biopsy and the resection). When inadequate, this can contribute to margin-positive primary resections and the need for reexcision for residual disease in as many as 39% to 87% of patients subsequently seen at tertiary care centers.[24] A combination of CT and MRI are used in preoperative planning. Contrary to other tumors in which chest radiograph may be adequate for assessing pulmonary metastases, chest CT is typically indicated for ruling out pulmonary disease in STS. CT of the abdomen and pelvis is used to characterize retroperitoneal STS. No studies have compared CT and MRI in retroperitoneal STS. However, double-contrast CT of the abdomen and pelvis is most commonly used to identify liver metastases, define vital structures that might require en bloc resection, and identify surrounding organs at risk for radiation exposure.[25]

MRI plays a central role in STS management and planning, particularly for structures affected by motion artifact, such as the extremities.[26] MRI is capable of producing images in a variety of planes and often has more familiar surgical, anatomic, or conventional radiographic orientations. Several authors have compared CT with MRI in the evaluation of extremity STS and have shown MRI to be superior in delineation between tumor and muscle, vessels, fat, and bone, but not between tumor and nerve.[27] Overall, MRI seems to be better for extremity STS. Multiple studies have also shown MRI to have superior accuracy for predicting STS resectability compared with CT.[28] MRI is also superior to CT in identifying muscle compartment invasion by the sarcoma, leading to improved clinical staging.[26] Despite most studies favoring MRI over CT, CT was found to be equivalent to MRI by the Radiation Diagnostic Oncology Group (RDOG). The RDOG prospectively studied 133 patients with primary STS across several institutions and found that CT was equivalent to MRI for determining involvement of muscle, bone, joint, and neurovasculature.[29] Therefore, CT is an excellent alternative in patients who cannot get an MRI, and should have similar ability to predict tumor invasion or help plan the operative strategy for limb-sparing resection in extremity STS.[21]

The role of PET scan for STS is still being examined and defined. It has been shown to correlate with STS grade and can be helpful for identifying distant metastases in patients with high-risk tumors. A recent study from Germany using 18(F)-fluorodeoxyglucose (FDG)-PET showed that tumor glycolytic phenotype (standardized uptake value [SUV]) correlated significantly with histologic grade, as determined by both the Fédération Nationale des Centres de Lutte Contre le Cancer (FNCLCC) and two-tier (high vs low) grading systems.[30] PET/CT has also been shown to be accurate and sensitive for detecting lymph node and bony metastases.[31] Finally, FDG-PET has been used to determine response to neoadjuvant chemotherapy for stratifying histopathologic response in patients with high-grade sarcomas.[32]

DIAGNOSTIC BIOPSY

Orientation of the STS biopsy is critical for preoperative planning in that the trajectory and scar should be parallel to the long axis of the extremity and lie within the area of subsequent en bloc tumor resection. Fine-needle aspiration (FNA) biopsy is classically described using a 21-gauge needle and a 10-mL syringe with several passes through the tissue and stained with Giemsa, Papanicolaou, and hematoxylin-eosin stains.[33] At select major sarcoma centers, FNA biopsy is frequently used for diagnostic purposes. Tertiary care institutions report 89% sensitivity in detecting malignancy, with 95% accuracy in grading when using FNA.[34] However, the accuracy of FNA biopsy is directly related to the skill and experience of the pathologist interpreting the sample.

Diagnostic percutaneous core needle biopsy is safe and reliable, and can be performed with local anesthesia for palpable masses or in conjunction with CT, ultrasound, or MRI for deep-seated tumors. Core needle biopsy can determine the STS histologic subtype and grade. Its main advantage over FNA biopsy is that it provides the pathologist with the histologic architecture of the tumor, which is often critical for diagnosing STS. Diagnostic accuracy of core needle biopsy is 95% to 99% compared with incisional biopsy.[35] Other groups propose using a combination of FNA and core needle biopsies to improve diagnostic accuracy (77% positive identification of subtype and 90% positive identification of grade) and efficiency, nearly eliminating the need for incisional biopsy.[36]

STS GRADING SYSTEMS

Grading should be assigned to all STSs, whenever possible. A few STSs are inherently nongradable, such as epithelioid sarcoma, alveolar soft part sarcoma, and clear cell sarcoma. Histologic grade is the strongest predictor of patient outcome of all of the known prognostic factors. However, controversy exists over which grading system to use, because no universally accepted standard exists. The AJCC adopted a three-grade system in the seventh edition,[37] compared with the traditional four-grade system.

STS grading incorporates differentiation, mitotic rate, and extent of necrosis. Alternate grading systems exist in the literature, such as the original Broders grading system introduced in the 1920s and the Markhede system introduced in the 1980s. The Broders system is based on degree of cellularity, nuclear atypia, necrosis, and mitotic rate, and is classified into four levels (I, II, III, IV), with grade I representing highly differentiated tumors and grade IV representing the other extreme.[38,39] Currently, the two most widely used grading systems are the FNCLCC (**Table 3**)[40] and National

Table 3
FNCLCC grading system

Tumor Differentiation	
Score 1	Sarcomas closely resemble normal adult mesenchymal tissue (eg, well-differentiated liposarcoma)
Score 2	Sarcomas in which histologic subtyping is defined (eg, myxoid liposarcoma)
Score 3	Embryonal and undifferentiated sarcomas (eg, synovial sarcomas, osteosarcomas, PNET)
Mitotic count	
Score 1	0–9 mitoses per 10 HPF
Score 2	10–19 mitoses per 10 HPF
Score 3	≥20 mitoses per 10 HPF
Tumor necrosis	
Score 0	No necrosis
Score 1	<50% tumor necrosis
Score 2	≥50% tumor necrosis
Histologic grade	
Grade 1	Total score 2–3
Grade 2	Total score 3–4
Grade 3	Total score 6–8

Differentiation Score According to Histologic Type	
Well-differentiated liposarcoma	1
Myxoid liposarcoma	2
Round cell liposarcoma	3
Pleomorphic liposarcoma	3
Well-differentiated fibrosarcoma	1
Conventional fibrosarcoma	2
Poorly differentiated fibrosarcoma	3
Myxofibrosarcoma	2
Pleomorphic MFH with storiform pattern	2
Pleomorphic MFH without storiform pattern	3
Giant cell MFH	3
Well-differentiated leiomyosarcoma	1
Conventional leiomyosarcoma	2
Poorly differentiated leiomyosarcoma	3
Embryonal/alveolar/pleomorphic rhabdomyosarcoma	3
Mesenchymal chondrosarcoma	3
Osteosarcoma	3
PNET	3
Malignant triton tumor	3
Synovial sarcoma	3
Well-differentiated angiosarcoma	2
Poorly differentiated/epithelioid angiosarcoma	3
Epithelioid sarcoma	3
Clear cell sarcoma	3

Abbreviations: HPF, high-power field; MFH, Malignant fibrous histiocytoma; PNET, pancreatic neuroendocrine tumor.

Data from Petterson H, Gillepsy T III, Hamlin DJ, et al. Primary musculoskeletal tumors: examination with MR imaging compared with conventional modalities. Radiology 1987;164(1):237–41; and Coindre JM. Grading of soft tissue sarcomas: review and update. Arch Pathol Lab Med 2006;130(10):1448–53; *Modified from* Guillou L, Coindre JM, Bonichon F, et al. Comparative study of the National Cancer Institute and French Federation of Cancer Centers Sarcoma Group grading systems in a population of 410 adult patients with soft tissue sarcoma. J Clin Oncol 1997;15:350–62; and Trojani M, Contesso G, Coindre JM, et al. Soft-tissue sarcomas of adults; study of pathological prognostic variables and definition of a histopathological grading system. Int J Cancer 1984;33(1):37–42.

Cancer Institute (NCI) systems (**Table 4**),[41] which are both three-grade systems. The FNCLCC grade is determined through differentiation (histology-specific; score of 1–3), mitotic activity (score of 1–3), and extent of necrosis (score of 0–2). The scores are summed to designate grade, with an overall score of 2 to 3 equivalent to grade 1; 4 to 5 indicating grade 2/intermediate-grade; and 6 to 8 indicating grade 3. Tumor differentiation is the most variable and subjective aspect of the FNCLCC system. However, it is also influential in that any sarcoma assigned a differentiation score of 3 will be at least intermediate- or high-grade on final calculation.[10] Certain types of sarcomas are assigned a differentiation score of 3, namely synovial sarcomas, embryonal sarcomas, undifferentiated sarcomas, and sarcomas of unknown/doubtful tumor type. Differentiation takes into account the histologic type and subtypes. For example, alveolar rhabdomyosarcoma and extraskeletal Ewing sarcoma are always considered high-grade, whereas well-differentiated liposarcoma and dermatofibrosarcoma protuberans (DFSP) are considered low-grade. Mitotic count is based on number of mitoses per 10 high-power fields (HPFs) with a score of 1 for 0 to 9 mitoses versus 3 for 20 or more mitoses.

In contrast to the FNCLCC system, the NCI system uses percentage of tumor necrosis and mitoses per HPF to divide STS into three categories. Grade 1 tumors tend to be well-differentiated, whereas grade 2 STSs have less than 15% of the surface area showing necrosis, and fewer than 5 mitoses per HPF. Grade 3 tumors have greater than 15% necrosis and more than 5 mitoses per HPF.

In general, grading is difficult and has its limitations. Grading is considered somewhat subjective, in that expert pathologists may disagree by as much as 30% on grade classification when blinded to the same specimens.[42] In accordance with the College of American Pathologists recommendations, the French system is preferred over the NCI system for reproducibility and slightly superior performance.[43,44]

Table 4
The National Cancer Institute grading system for soft tissue sarcomas

Common Histologic Types		
Grade 1	Grade 2	Grade 3
Well-differentiated liposarcoma	Pleomorphic liposarcoma	Alveolar rhabdomyosarcoma
Myxoid liposarcoma	Fibrosarcoma	Soft tissue osteosarcoma
Deep-seated dermatofibrosarcoma protuberans	Malignant fibrous histiocytoma	Primitive neuroectodermal tumor
Some leiomyosarcomas	Malignant hemangiopericytoma	Alveolar soft part sarcoma
Epithelioid hemangioendothelioma	Synovial sarcoma	Mesenchymal chondrosarcoma
Spindle cell hemangioendothelioma	Leiomyosarcoma	
Infantile fibrosarcoma	Neurofibrosarcoma	
Subcutaneous myxofibrosarcoma		
	or 0%–15% necrosis	or >15% necrosis

Adapted from Brown FM, Fletcher CD. Problems in grading soft tissue sarcomas. Am J Clin Pathol 2000;114(Suppl):S82–9; and data from Bland KI, McCoy DM, Kinard RE, et al. Application of magnetic resonance imaging and computerized tomography as an adjunct to the surgical management of soft tissue sarcomas. Ann Surg 1987;205(5):473–81.

Accurate grading from core needle biopsies, especially when neoadjuvant chemo-therapy or radiation will be administered, can be extremely difficult because of alterations in nuclear features, mitotic activity, cellularity, and induced necrosis. Targeting image-guided core needle biopsies to avoid an area of obvious necrosis can increase viable tumor yield for appropriate grading.[45] Sampling error is another issue, especially with large tumors. Other tumors appear cellular and mitotically active but behave in a clinically low-grade fashion, such as congenital/infantile fibrosarcoma. Finally, in certain sarcomas the histologic subtype in effect defines behavior so that grade becomes redundant (eg, well-differentiated liposarcoma, considered low-grade; alveolar rhabdomyosarcoma, considered high-grade), whereas other subtypes are historically considered ungradable (eg, epithelioid sarcoma, clear cell sarcoma, and alveolar soft part sarcoma) or not entirely useful (eg, angiosarcomas).

STS STAGING SYSTEMS

Currently two staging systems are used for STS, which complicates institutional comparisons: the AJCC/International Union Against Cancer and the Enneking staging system of the Musculoskeletal Tumor Society (MSTS).[46] The MSTS system, which only subdivides sarcomas into low- and high-grade, defines stages according to grade, compartmental status (intracompartmental or extracompartmental), and presence or absence of metastases (**Table 5**). The AJCC staging system is the most widely accepted system worldwide. It dates back to the fourth edition published in 1992,[47] with three subsequent revisions, culminating in the most recent seventh edition.[24] N1 disease was reclassified as stage III in the seventh edition. The grading system was also reformatted into a three-grade system. Lesions of "uncertain malignant potential," such as Kaposi's sarcoma, DFSP, desmoid tumors, and sarcoma arising from dura mater, brain, parenchymatous organs, or hollow viscera, are no longer included. Finally, the seventh edition of AJCC placed gastrointestinal stromal tumors (GIST) into a separate staging system (**Table 6**).

The AJCC staging system is broken down into T, N, and M categories. T stage reflects the size of the tumor, which influences distant metastatic-free and overall survival rates. T1 tumors are 5 cm or less and T2 are greater than 5 cm. There are also *a* and *b* location designations, with *a* signifying superficial tumors (lack of involvement of the superficial investing muscular fascia) and *b* representing deep tumors

Table 5
Musculoskeletal Tumor Society surgical staging system

Stage	Grade	Local Extent	Metastasis
I-A	Low	Intracompartmental	None
I-B	Low	Extracompartmental	None
II-A	High	Intracompartmental	None
II-B	High	Extracompartmental	None
III	Any	Any	Present

Intracompartmental tumors are confined within the boundaries of well-defined anatomic structures (functional muscle group, joint, subcutis). Extracompartmental neoplasms arise within or involve extrafascial spaces or planes and do not have natural anatomic barriers to extension.

Data from Enneking WF, Spanier SS, Goodman MA. A system for surgical staging of musculoskeletal sarcoma. Clin Orthop Relat Res 1980;153:106–20; and Tateishi U, Kawai A, Chuman H, et al. PET/CT allows stratification of responders to neoadjuvant chemotherapy for high-grade sarcoma: a prospective study. Clin Nucl Med 2011;36(7):526–32.

Table 6
AJCC staging system, 7th edition

Stage	Grade	Tumor	Node	Metastasis
IA	G1–GX	T1a–b	N0	M0
IB	G1–GX	T2a–b	N0	M0
IIA	G2–G3	T1a–b	N0	M0
IIB	G2	T2a–b	N0	M0
III	G3	T2a–b	N0	M0
	Any G	Any T	N1	M0
IV	Any G	Any T	Any N	M1

T1, ≤5 cm; T2, >5 cm; a, superficial; b, deep.
Data from Noria S, Davis A, Kandel R, et al. Residual disease following unplanned excision of soft tissue sarcoma of an extremity. J Bone Joint Surg Am 1996;78(5):650–5.

(deep to or involving the superficial fascia, all retroperitoneal STSs). Lymph node involvement (N1) is also a prognostic factor for overall survival. Recent studies suggest that nodal involvement is less ominous than distant metastases.[48,49] Whether sentinel lymph node biopsy has a role in STS histologies prone to metastasize to lymph nodes, namely epithelioid or synovial sarcoma, is still a matter of debate.[50] Regardless of T or N status, the presence of metastatic (M1) disease signifies stage IV assignment and is the single strongest predictor of survival.[12]

ADDITIONAL PROGNOSTIC FACTORS

There are additional prognostic factors that the current AJCC seventh edition STS staging system does not incorporate, including primary tumor site, patient age, resection margin status, molecular staging/prognosis markers, the ongoing effect of size for tumors greater than 5 cm, and whether the tumor is primary versus recurrent.[12] The site of the primary tumor influences 5-year survival and can also place anatomic constraints on the ability to perform a negative margin resection. Estimates of 5-year overall survival rates for retroperitoneal and head and neck STSs are fairly low at 25% to 55%, even at major STS centers, compared with 60% to 75% for high-risk stage III extremity STS.[12] Data from a study at MD Anderson Cancer Center (MDACC) involving 402 patients with relapsed STS showed that the site of the primary tumor and the locally recurrent status have implications on STS-specific survival rates; 5-year survival for extremity/superficial truncal STS was 55% versus 16% for head and neck/deep truncal STS.[51]

As discussed in more detail in another article by Kotilingam and colleagues elsewhere in this issue, STS resection margin status is another prognostic factor of importance, not currently accounted for in the AJCC staging system. In a 2002 retrospective study of more than 2000 patients, researchers at Memorial Sloan-Kettering Cancer Center noted that STS disease-specific survival for STS was significantly better for margin-negative resections.[52] The 5-year disease-specific survival rates for negative versus positive margins were 83% and 75%, respectively. In addition, MDACC confirmed the importance of negative resection margins for stage III disease, with a 5-year survival of 88% versus 71% for margin positive/margin uncertain resections.[53] A recently published study by MDACC emphasized the importance of surgical margins in retroperitoneal STS resection and the association with local recurrence and death.[54]

A primary tumor versus locally recurrent tumor status is important in that previous local recurrence is a major risk factor for future recurrences. One report studied 753 patients with intermediate- and high-grade extremity STS at a single institution and found that the single greatest risk factor for future recurrence was a prior local recurrence.[55] In this study, local recurrence was also the most significant factor associated with decreased STS-specific survival; patients with a local recurrence were three times more likely to die of STS than patients who were recurrence-free. Similar findings were noted by MDACC in a larger study of 1225 patients with localized STS, in which local recurrence predicted future recurrences.[12] These findings are probably a testament to the biologic aggressiveness of the tumor.

One additional prognostic factor that is not highlighted in the current AJCC staging system is size of STS beyond 5 cm. Any primary STS greater than 5 cm is designated as T2 in the current staging system. The Royal Marsden group analyzed 316 patients with previously untreated STS treated at their institution and found that both margin status and a tumor size greater than 15 cm statistically impacted disease-specific survival and, therefore, prognosis.[56]

THE FUTURE/CONCLUSIONS

The future of STS staging will likely incorporate specific molecular markers that will impact grading systems. Both genomic and proteomic analysis and tissue microarray analysis will become useful for revising staging systems and the ability to predict disease progression, treatment response, and survival.[57] Numerous candidate molecular markers of STS aid in histopathologic diagnosis; however, data are insufficient to include them within the current staging system. Specific genetic alterations can be further subclassified by their mechanism. For example, Ewing sarcoma is the result of a reciprocal translocation resulting in an oncogenic fusion transcript (Ewing sarcoma breakpoint region 1 and Friend leukemia virus integration 1 [EWSR1-FLI1]), whereas specific oncogene mutations in c-kit and platelet-derived growth factor receptor A (PDGFRA) give rise to GIST. Specific molecular markers that have been shown to have potential importance in STS prognosis include p53,[23] Ki-67,[58] PDGFR-α,[59] ß-catenin,[60] c-kit,[44] and Skp2.[61]

The paradigm of understanding of the molecular pathogenesis of STS continues to shift as molecular profiling evolves. For example, leiomyosarcoma and pleomorphic liposarcoma were previously thought to display multiple, complex karyotypic abnormalities with no specific pattern.[62] However, a recent publication discovered distinct molecular subtypes of leiomyosarcoma using molecular profiling. In addition, expression of certain mRNA (ACTG2, CASQ2, SLMAP, CFL2, MYLK) was associated with disease-specific survival.[63] Integrative genomic characterization and staging systems are emerging for GIST, leiomyosarcoma, and synovial sarcoma that have prognostic and potential therapeutic implications.[64]

In summary, STS staging is a constantly evolving process, as evident by the multiple revisions to the AJCC staging system, most recently updated in the seventh edition. Although the AJCC staging system for STS is the most widely accepted worldwide, other staging systems exist. Oncologic orthopedic surgeons still favor the MSTS staging system. Grading is still of utmost importance and has been adapted into a three-tier system. Besides STS, another category of soft tissue tumors is labeled tumors of intermediate malignancy (although not included as bona fide sarcomas), which have low to modest rates of local recurrence and a poorly defined capacity for distant metastases. These tumors include epithelioid hemangioendothelioma, composite hemangioendothelioma, plexiform fibrohistiocytic tumor, and angiomatoid fibrous histiocytoma. Although rare, these tumors continue to pose a challenge to treatment and prognostication. The STS most difficult to categorize are those with uncertain malignant potential, such as solitary fibrous tumors, GIST, and glomus tumors, some of which have developed completely separate staging systems and may not even be considered sarcomas.

Beyond the current TNM staging system, a multitude of prognostic factors for STS will continue to be discovered and ultimately incorporated into future revisions of the staging system. Molecular staging, through discovery of new oncogenic mutations and genetic profiling, will strongly impact STS prognosis and, ultimately, treatment recommendations and outcomes. The goal is for discovery of molecular markers in STS that can be directly tested for in patients with known clinical outcomes, thereby determining whether any of these can be incorporated into future STS systems.

REFERENCES

1. Jemal A, Siegel R, Ward E, et al. Cancer Statistics 2009. CA Cancer J Clin 2009; 59:225–49.
2. Cancer facts and figures 2010. American Cancer Society Web site. Available at: http://www.cancer.org/acs/groups/content/@epidemiologysurveilance/documents/document/acspc-026238.pdf. Accessed May 27, 2011.
3. Heslin MJ, Lewis JJ, Nadler E, et al. Prognostic factors associated with long-term survival for retroperitoneal sarcoma: implications for management. J Clin Oncol 1997;15(8):2832–9.
4. Mendenhall WM, Zlotecki RA, Hochwald SN, et al. Retroperitoneal soft tissue sarcoma. Cancer 2005;104(4):669–75.
5. Brennan MF, Singer S, Maki RG. Sarcomas of the soft tissue and bone. In: DeVita VT Jr, Hellman S, Rosenberg SA, editors. Principles and practice of oncology, Vols. 1 and 2, 8th edition. Philadelphia: Lippincott Williams & Wilkins; 2008. p. 1741–833.
6. Lewis JJ, Leung D, Woodruff JM, et al. Retroperitoneal soft-tissue sarcoma: analysis of 500 patients treated and followed at a single institution. Ann Surg 1998; 228(3):355–65.
7. Russell WO. The pathologic diagnosis of cancer–a crescendo of importance in current and future therapies. Ward Burdick Award Lecture. Am J Clin Pathol 1980;73(1):3–11.
8. Russel WO, Cohen J, Enzinger FM, et al. A clinical and pathological staging system for soft tissue sarcomas. Cancer 1977;40:1562.
9. Cormier JM, Pollock RE. Soft tissue sarcomas. CA Cancer J Clin 2004;54: 94–109.
10. Coindre JM, Terrier P, Guillou L, et al. Predictive value of grade for metastasis development in the main histologic types of adult soft tissue sarcomas: a study of 1240 patients from the French Federation of Cancer Centers Sarcoma Group. Cancer 2001;91:1914–26.
11. Fong Y, Coit DG, Woodruff JM, et al. Lymph node metastasis from soft tissue sarcoma in adults. Analysis of data from a prospective database of 1772 sarcoma patients. Ann Surg 1993;217:72–7.
12. Kotilingam D, Lev DC, Lazar AJ, et al. Staging soft tissue sarcoma: evolution and change. CA Cancer J Clin 2006;56:282–91.
13. Brady MS, Gaynor JJ, Brennan MF. Radiation-induced sarcoma of bone and soft tissue. Arch Surg 1992;127:1379.
14. Zahm SH, Faumeni JF Jr. The epidemiology of soft tissue sarcoma. Semin Oncol 1997;24:504–14.
15. Hardell L, Sandstron A. A case-control study: soft tissue sarcoma and exposure to phenoxyacetic acids or chlorophenols. Br J Cancer 1979;39:711–7.

16. Smith AH, Pearce NE, Fisher DO. Soft tissue sarcoma and exposure to phenox-yherbicides and chlorophenols in New Zealand. J Natl Cancer Inst 1984;73:1111.
17. Golshan M, Smith B. Prevention and management of arm lymphedema in the patient with breast cancer. J Support Oncol 2006;4(8):381–6.
18. Muller R, Hajdu SI, Brennan MF. Lymphangiosarcoma associated with chronic filarial lymphedema. Cancer 1987;59:179.
19. Levine EA. Prognostic factors in soft tissue sarcoma. Semin Surg Oncol 1999;17: 23–32.
20. Vorburger SA, Hunt KK. Experimental approaches. In: Pollock RE, editor. Soft tissue sarcomas. Hamilton, Ontario (Canada): BC Decker, Inc; 2002. p. 89–109.
21. Borden EC, Baker LH, Bell RS, et al. Soft tissue sarcomas of adults: state of the translational science. Clin Cancer Res 2003;9:1941–56.
22. Latres E, Drobnjak M, Pollack D, et al. Chromosome 17 abnormalities and TP53 mutations in adult soft tissue sarcomas. Am J Pathol 1994;145:345–55.
23. Hieken TJ, Das Gupta TK. Mutant p53 expression: a marker of diminished survival in well-differentiated soft tissue sarcoma. Clin Cancer Res 1996;2:1391–5.
24. Noria S, Davis A, Kandel R, et al. Residual disease following unplanned excision of soft tissue sarcoma of an extremity. J Bone Joint Surg Am 1996;78(5):650–5.
25. Tzeng CW, Smith JK, Heslin MJ. Soft tissue sarcoma: preoperative and postop-erative imaging for staging. Surg Oncol Clin N Am 2007;16:389–402.
26. Demas BE, Heelan RT, Lane J, et al. Soft-tissue sarcomas of the extremities: comparison of MR and CT in determining the extent of disease. AJR Am J Roent-genol 1988;150(3):615–20.
27. Pettersson H, Gillespy T III, Hamlin DJ, et al. Primary musculoskeletal tumors: examination with MR imaging compared with conventional modalities. Radiology 1987;164(1):237–41.
28. Bland KI, McCoy DM, Kinard RE, et al. Application of magnetic resonance imaging and computerized tomography as an adjunct to the surgical manage-ment of soft tissue sarcomas. Ann Surg 1987;205(5):473–81.
29. Panick DM, Gatsonis C, Rosenthal DI, et al. CT and MR imaging in the local staging of primary malignant musculoskeletal neoplasms: report of the Radiology Diagnostic Oncology Group. Radiology 1997;202(1):237–46.
30. Benz MR, Dry SM, Eilber FC, et al. Correlation between glycolytic phenotype and tumor grade in soft-tissue sarcomas by 18F-FDG PET. J Nucl Med 2010;51(8): 1174–81.
31. Benz MR, Tcheckmedyian N, Eilber FC, et al. Utilization of positron emission tomography in the management of patients with sarcoma. Curr Opin Oncol 2009;21(4):345–51.
32. Tateishi U, Kawai A, Chuman H, et al. PET/CT allows stratification of responders to neoadjuvant chemotherapy for high-grade sarcoma: a prospective study. Clin Nucl Med 2011;36(7):526–32.
33. Tong TR, Chow T, Chan OW, et al. Clear-cell sarcoma diagnosis by fine-needle aspiration: cytologic, histologic, and ultrastructural features; potential pitfalls; and literature review. Diagn Cytopathol 2002;26:174–80.
34. Ng VY, Thomas K, Crist M, et al. Fine needle aspiration for clinical triage of extremity soft tissue masses. Clin Orthop Relat Res 2010;468(4):1120–8.
35. Heslin MJ, Lewis JJ, Woodruff JM, et al. Core needle biopsy for diagnosis of extremity soft tissue sarcoma. Ann Surg Oncol 1997;4:425–31.
36. Domanski HA, Akerman M, Carlén B, et al. Core-needle biopsy performed by the cytopathologist: a technique to complement fine-needle aspiration of soft tissue and bone lesions. Cancer 2005;105(4):229–39.

37. Edge SB, Byrd DR, Compton CC, et al, editors. Soft tissue sarcoma. AJCC Cancer Staging Manual. 7th edition. New York: Springer; 2010.
38. Broders A, Hargrave R, Meyerding HW. Pathological features of soft tissue fibrosarcoma with special reference to the grading of its malignancy. Surg Gynecol Obstet 1939;69:267–80.
39. Coindre JM, Trojani M, Contesso G, et al. Reproducibility of a histopathological grading system for adult soft tissue sarcoma. Cancer 1986;58:306–9.
40. Coindre JM. Grading of soft tissue sarcomas: review and update. Arch Pathol Lab Med 2006;130(10):1448–53.
41. Brown FM, Fletcher CD. Problems in grading soft tissue sarcomas. Am J Clin Pathol 2000;114(Suppl):S82–9.
42. Deyrup AT, Weiss SW. Grading of soft tissue sarcomas: the challenge of providing precise information in an imprecise world. Histopathology 2006;48:42–50.
43. Guillou L, Coindre JM, Bonichon F, et al. Comparative study of the National Cancer Institute and French Federation of Cancer Centers Sarcoma Group grading systems in a population of 410 adult patients with soft tissue sarcoma. J Clin Oncol 1997;15:350–62.
44. Rubin BP, Fletcher CD, Inwards C, et al. Protocol for the examination of specimens from patients with soft tissue tumors of indeterminate malignant potential, malignant soft tissue tumors, and borderline/locally aggressive and malignant bone tumors. Arch Pathol Lab Med 2006;130(11):1616–29.
45. Narvani AA, Tsiridis E, Saifuddin A, et al. Does image guidance improve accuracy of core needle biopsy in diagnosis of soft tissue tumours? Acta Orthop Belg 2009; 75(2):239–44.
46. Enneking WF, Spanier SS, Goodman MA. A system for surgical staging of musculoskeletal sarcoma. Clin Orthop Relat Res 1980;153:106–20.
47. Beahrs OH, Hensen DE, Hunter RV, et al. Manual for staging of cancer. 4th edition. Philadelphia: JB Lippincott; 1992.
48. Riad S, Griffin AM, Liberman B, et al. Lymph node metastasis in soft tissue sarcoma in an extremity. Clin Orthop Relat Res 2004;(426):129–34.
49. Behranwala KA, A'Hern R, Omar AM, et al. Prognosis of lymph node metastasis in soft tissue sarcoma. Ann Surg Oncol 2004;11:714–9.
50. Blazer DG III, Sabel MS, Sondak VK. Is there a role for sentinel lymph node biopsy in the management of sarcoma? Surg Oncol 2003;12:201–6.
51. Zagars GK, Ballo MT, Pisters PW, et al. Prognostic factors for disease-specific survival after first relapse of soft-tissue sarcoma: analysis of 402 patients with disease relapse after initial conservative surgery and radiotherapy. Int J Radiat Oncol Biol Phys 2003;57:739–47.
52. Stojadinovic A, Leung DH, Hoos A, et al. Analysis of the prognostic significance of microscopic margins in 2,084 localized primary adult soft tissue sarcomas. Ann Surg 2002;235:424–34.
53. Zagars GK, Ballo MT, Pisters PW, et al. Prognostic factors for patients with localized soft-tissue sarcoma treated with conservation surgery and radiation therapy: an analysis of 225 patients. Cancer 2003;97:2530–43.
54. Anaya DA, Lev DC, Pollock RE. The role of surgical margin status in retroperitoneal sarcoma. J Surg Oncol 2008;98:607–10.
55. Eilber FC, Rosen G, Nelson SD, et al. High-grade extremity soft tissue sarcomas: factors predictive of local recurrence and its effect on morbidity and mortality. Ann Surg 2003;237:218–26.
56. Ramanathan RC, A'Hern R, Fisher C, et al. Modified staging system for extremity soft tissue sarcomas. Ann Surg Oncol 1999;6:57–69.

57. Packeisen J, Korsching E, Herbst H, et al. Demystified...tissue microarray technology. Mol Pathol 2003;56:198–204.
58. Hoos A, Stojadinovic A, Mastorides S, et al. High Ki-67 proliferative index predicts disease specific survival in patients with high-risk soft tissue sarcomas. Cancer 2001;92:869–74.
59. Lopez-Guerrero JA, Navarro S, Noguera R, et al. Mutational analysis of the c-KIT and PDGFRalpha in a series of molecularly well-characterized synovial sarcomas. Diagn Mol Pathol 2005;14:134–9.
60. Kuhnen C, Herter P, Muller O, et al. Beta-catenin in soft tissue sarcomas: expression is related to proliferative activity in high-grade sarcomas. Mod Pathol 2000; 13:1005–13.
61. Huan HY, Kang HY, Li CF, et al. Skp2 overexpression is highly representative of intrinsic biological aggressiveness and independently associated with poor prognosis in primary localized myxofibrosarcomas. Clin Cancer Res 2006;12:487–98.
62. Jain S, Xu R, Prieto VG, et al. Molecular classification of soft tissue sarcomas and its clinical applications. Int J Clin Exp Pathol 2010;3(4):416–28.
63. Beck AH, Lee CH, Witten DM, et al. Discovery of molecular subtypes in leiomyosarcoma through integrative molecular profiling. Oncogene 2010;29(6):1–18.
64. Ylipää A, Hunt KK, Yang J, et al. Integrative genomic characterization and a genomic staging system for gastrointestinal stromal tumors. Cancer 2011; 117(2):380–9.

Modern Surgical Therapy: Limb Salvage and the Role of Amputation for Extremity Soft-Tissue Sarcomas

Marco L. Ferrone, MD[a], Chandrajit P. Raut, MD, MSc[b],*

KEYWORDS

- Extremity sarcoma • Limb salvage • Radiation therapy
- Limb infusion/limb perfusion

Approximately 50% of sarcomas arise in the extremities, with a threefold higher rate observed in the lower extremities than in the upper extremities.[1] Historically the surgical management of extremity soft-tissue sarcomas (ESTS) commonly involved amputation. However, radical surgery was not necessarily curative. In an early series of 297 patients with lower extremity ESTS from Memorial Sloan-Kettering Cancer Center, 47% underwent amputation.[2] While local recurrence rates were higher in patients undergoing en bloc wide soft-tissue resection, the 5- and 10-year overall survival (OS) rates were 63% and 50% after limb-sparing surgery and 45% and 29% after amputation. Such results led investigators to seek to improve local control with less morbid surgery.

Limb-sparing, function-preserving surgery is now the standard of care for ESTS. Adjuvant therapies such as radiation therapy (RT) and chemotherapy are used selectively in an effort to minimize both local recurrence and distant spread. Less common modalities, such as isolated limb perfusion (ILP), isolated limb infusion (ILI), and hyperthermia are being evaluated to potentially expand the cohort of individuals who may be eligible for limb-sparing surgery and to improve outcomes. This article reviews the standard and evolving approaches to the management of ESTS.

The authors have nothing to disclose.

[a] Department of Orthopedics, Brigham and Women's Hospital, Center for Sarcoma and Bone Oncology, Dana-Farber Cancer Institute, Harvard Medical School, 75 Francis Street, Boston, MA 02115, USA

[b] Department of Surgery, Brigham and Women's Hospital, Center for Sarcoma and Bone Oncology, Dana-Farber Cancer Institute, Harvard Medical School, 75 Francis Street, Boston, MA 02115, USA

* Corresponding author.

E-mail address: craut@partners.org

Surg Oncol Clin N Am 21 (2012) 201–213
doi:10.1016/j.soc.2011.11.001
1055-3207/12/$ – see front matter © 2012 Elsevier Inc. All rights reserved.

RISK FACTORS FOR RECURRENCE AND DEATH

In a large contemporary retrospective review of 997 ESTS from Istituto Nazionale Tumori in Milan, Italy, margin status, size, grade, depth, and histologic subtype were independent predictors of mortality.[3] The 5- and 10-year mortality estimates were 16% and 19% for patients with macroscopically complete resections with negative microscopic margins (R0 resection), and 29% and 38% for patients with macroscopically complete resections with positive (<1 mm) microscopic margins (R1 resection) (P = .0003). Among the R0 patients, cause of death was distant metastases in 100% whereas among R1 patients, 17% died of locoregional progression without distant metastases. Among the subset of patients with R1 resections, the 5- and 10-year mortality rates were 21% and 21% for those with a biological margin (such as intact fascia) compared with 30% and 40% for those with tumor directly at the inked margin (P = .36). Additional risk factors negatively affecting local recurrence-free survival (LRFS), distant recurrence-free survival (DRFS), and disease-specific survival (DSS) included patient age older than 50 years, recurrent sarcoma, and proximal location.[4]

Individuals diagnosed with or suspected of having ESTS should be referred to centers specializing in the management of such tumors. Treatment at such centers improves both limb salvage and survival rates.[5]

LIMB-SALVAGE SURGERY

The definitive therapy for ESTS, as for all localized sarcomas, is a radical, margin-negative resection (**Fig. 1**). No adjuvant or neoadjuvant therapy can substitute for an inadequate operation.[6] When margins are believed to be either microscopically positive (R1 resection) or macroscopically positive (R2 resection), one must strongly consider whether another operation is warranted to achieve sufficient margins.

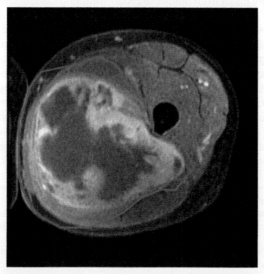

Fig. 1. Contrast-enhanced magnetic resonance imaging (MRI) of proximal left thigh high-grade malignant peripheral nerve sheath tumor after neoadjuvant radiation therapy. The operation required a radical en bloc resection of the medial compartment of the thigh. The sciatic nerve and the posterior compartment were spared, although the fascia of the anterior and posterior compartments was resected medially. The periosteum of the adjacent portion of the femur was removed en bloc with the tumor.

What constitutes an adequate margin still remains a matter of debate, dependent in part on histology and tumor location. In general, a 1- to 2-cm margin of normal, non-neoplastic tissue should be the goal of any operation. However, a close margin in the setting of an intact fascial plane is usually acceptable. When such a margin cannot be achieved because of proximity or involvement of critical neurovascular structures, RT, ILP/ILI, and resection of vascular and/or neural structures with reconstruction should be considered (**Fig. 2**).

As discussed herein, RT is commonly used to reduce the risk of local recurrence while sparing the limb and functionality even after a margin-negative resection. However, limb-sparing, function-preserving therapy does not always require RT. Patients with small, low-grade tumors resected completely or certain small, superficial high-grade tumors resected with wide margins may be treated with surgery alone. Furthermore, patients with certain histologic subtypes of ESTS, such as atypical lipomatous tumors, which have a low risk of local recurrence and distant spread, may be treated with surgery alone despite close margins.[7]

In patients with metastatic disease, surgery for the primary or a locally recurrent tumor may still be considered. The goal of surgery changes from curative intent to palliation. **Fig. 3** illustrates a patient with an unclassified sarcoma of the left popliteal fossa with regional soft-tissue and lung metastases, who underwent resection of the popliteal lesion for pain control. **Fig. 4** shows images of patient with a local recurrence in the right calf causing a fibular fracture and pain, requiring amputation even in the context of lung metastases.

RECONSTRUCTION

The ability to save a limb and retain function after resection of a sarcoma may require complex soft-tissue and neurovascular reconstruction. Reconstruction may be performed at the time of the original resection or may be staged after a short interval, particularly if there is concern about the margins. Although a comprehensive review

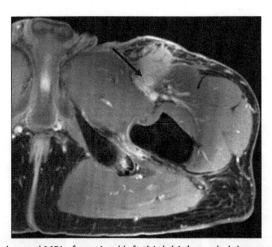

Fig. 2. Contrast-enhanced MRI of proximal left thigh high-grade leiomyosarcoma after neo-adjuvant radiation therapy. At the time of surgery, the superficial femoral artery (*arrow*) immediately deep to the tumor was resected en bloc with the tumor, the overlying skin and soft tissue, and sartorius muscle. The artery was replaced with a contralateral reversed saphenous vein graft. The soft-tissue defect was closed with a contralateral rectus abdominis myocutaneous flap.

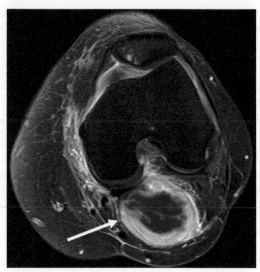

Fig. 3. Contrast-enhanced MRI of unclassified sarcoma of popliteal fossa (*arrow*). Although the patient had locoregional and distant metastases, resection of the primary site was required for symptomatic relief.

of reconstruction options is beyond the scope of this article, the oncologic surgeon should consider preoperatively the need for reconstruction. Split-thickness skin grafts, full-thickness skin grafts, rotational fasciocutaneous or myocutaneous flaps, pedicled muscle flaps, free flaps, nerve interpositions, and other advanced reconstructions by a plastic surgeon, and vascular grafts by a vascular surgeon, may be necessary.

RADIATION THERAPY

The landmark prospective phase III trial from the National Cancer Institute (NCI) randomizing patients with ESTS to limb-sparing surgery plus external beam radiation therapy (EBRT) or amputation established the current standard of care.[8] In this study, 27 patients underwent limb-sparing surgery plus EBRT (5000 rad to the anatomic area and 6000–7000 rad to the tumor bed), and 16 patients underwent amputation. All patients received postoperative chemotherapy. There were 4 local recurrences in

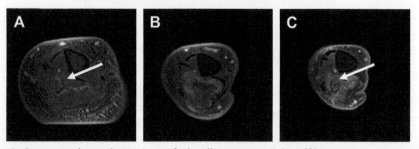

Fig. 4. Contrast-enhanced MRI views of a locally recurrent right calf leiomyosarcoma. Tumor appears to invade the anteromedial cortex of the fibula proximally (*A, arrow*) and distally (*C, arrow*). The mid portion of the fibula is completely replaced by tumor (*B*). Although the patient had undergoing multimodality therapy for lung metastases, an amputation was required because of intractable pain from the fibular fracture.

the limb-salvage group and none in the amputation group ($P = .06$). There were no differences in 5-year disease-free survival (DFS) (71% vs 78%, $P = .75$) or 5-year OS (83% vs 88%, $P = .99$). This trial established the new standard of care: radical resection plus EBRT has no worse long-term survival outcomes than amputation, while allowing limb preservation. However, EBRT following a marginal excision should not be considered an adequate substitute for a more radical function-sparing resection achieving wide margins.

Another prospective trial from the NCI randomized patients with ESTS treated with limb-sparing surgery (and for high-grade tumor patients only, postoperative adjuvant chemotherapy) to receive or not receive postoperative EBRT.[9] Among patients with high-grade ESTS, the estimated 10-year actuarial local failure rates were 0% in the EBRT arm and 22% in the no-EBRT arm ($P = .003$). There were no differences in distant recurrence or OS rates. Among patients with low-grade tumors (no chemotherapy), local recurrences were noted in 4% who received EBRT and 33% who did not ($P = .016$). When patients with desmoid tumors and dermatofibrosarcoma protuberans were excluded, the rates of local recurrence were 5% and 32%, respectively ($P = .067$).

Based on these data, the authors typically offer EBRT to patients undergoing limb-sparing surgery for large, deep tumors, high-grade tumors, tumors incompletely excised, and tumors lying close to neurovascular structures.

Are there patients in whom EBRT is not necessary? In a study of 74 patients with primary localized truncal and ESTS treated without RT at Brigham and Women's Hospital and Dana-Farber Cancer Institute, the 10-year actuarial local recurrence rate was 7% and the 10-year OS rate was 73%.[10] The only predictor of local recurrence was a histologic margin of less than 1 cm. Of interest, tumor grade was not a predictor of local recurrence. Of importance is that the median tumor size was 4 cm and one-third of the tumors were superficial, potentially reflecting a selection bias for the type of patients not treated with EBRT.

Based on these data, the authors offer the option of no RT for patients with small (<5 cm) tumors for which at least 1-cm margins are possible, particularly if the tumors are superficial, and provided that the patient can reliably be followed and that a local recurrence could still be treated with salvage function-sparing surgery. Although these data did not find a difference in local recurrence based on tumor grade, the authors are cautious about offering no radiation to patients with high grade tumors.

PREOPERATIVE VERSUS POSTOPERATIVE RADIATION THERAPY

Although the favorable impact of EBRT has been established, the timing of RT (preoperative, intraoperative, or postoperative) remains controversial. A Canadian phase III trial randomized 190 patients with ESTS to either preoperative EBRT (50 Gy in 25 fractions) or postoperative EBRT (66 Gy in 33 fractions).[11] Wound complication rates were higher in those treated with preoperative EBRT (35% vs 17%, $P = .01$); the largest number of wound complications was seen in patients with thigh sarcomas. Lower extremity location and tumor diameter greater than 10 cm were independent predictors of wound complications.

OS was better in those receiving preoperative EBRT, with 85% alive in the preoperative EBRT group versus 72% alive in the postoperative EBRT group at last contact ($P = .05$).[11] However, the excess number of deaths in the latter group appeared to derive from causes other than progression of sarcoma.

In the first 6 weeks after surgery, patients receiving preoperative EBRT had worse function by mean Musculoskeletal Tumor Society rating, Toronto Extremity Salvage

Score, and Short-Form-36 bodily pain score.[11] However, these differences disappeared at later time points. Moreover, a follow-up analysis of this study demonstrated that more patients had clinically significant fibrosis in the postoperative EBRT group than in the preoperative EBRT group (48% vs 32%, P = .07).[12] In turn, fibrosis adversely affected patient function at 2 years following treatment.

In the authors' institutional experience, significant predictors for wound complications in patients with extremity and truncal sarcomas treated with preoperative EBRT and radical resections included diabetes, large tumor size, and close tumor proximity to the skin (Baldini EH, Raut CP, unpublished data, November 2011). The authors continue to favor the use of preoperative EBRT because they are thus able to use a lower total treatment dose (50 Gy preoperatively vs 66 Gy postoperatively), but remain cognizant of the potential risk factors in planning how the resection bed will be closed or reconstructed. Furthermore, the preoperative EBRT field is contoured to encompass the visualized mass plus a margin, whereas postoperative treatment generally requires treatment of the entire operative bed usually with a 5-cm radial margin; the radiation field will also extend to the drain site. Thus, the preoperative approach enables treatment of a smaller field, an important consideration when fields may extend across a joint or potentially cover genitalia. Consequently, the potential benefits of preoperative EBRT include lower total radiation dose, smaller treatment fields, and better long-term functional outcomes. However, patients need to be counseled regarding the risks of wound complications.

BRACHYTHERAPY

Catheter-based brachytherapy (BT) may be used either alone or in combination with EBRT for the treatment of ESTS. In general, catheters are placed at the time of surgery across margins of concern and are sutured into place in the deep tissue with dissolvable sutures. Catheters are brought out through individual puncture sites in the skin, and secured into place (**Fig. 5**). Radioactive seeds are loaded into the catheters around postoperative day 5 (to allow sufficient time for wound healing).[13]

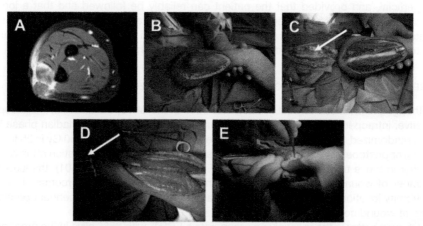

Fig. 5. Contrast-enhanced MRI image (*A*) and intraoperative photo (*B*) illustrate resection of a recurrent right forearm malignant peripheral nerve sheath tumor abutting the ulna, requiring radical resection of the lateral forearm tissue including the ulnar periosteum after preoperative external beam radiation therapy (*C, arrow*). Brachytherapy catheters were placed to further treat the bony margin (*D, arrow*) to minimize the risk of local recurrence without compromising limb function. Free flap reconstruction was required (*E*).

In the only reported prospective trial evaluating BT in soft-tissue sarcoma (STS), investigators at Memorial Sloan-Kettering Cancer Center randomized 164 patients with extremity or truncal STS to BT or no BT following R0/R1 resections.[14] Most patients had large, high-grade, primary tumors. With a median follow-up of 76 months, the local control rates in the BT arm was 82% versus 69% in the no-BT arm. Of importance, improved local control was noted only in patients with high-grade lesions (89% vs 66%, $P = .0025$). An earlier report from this same trial demonstrated overall and major complication rates of 44% and 22%, respectively, in the BT arm, and 14% and 3% in the no-BT arm.[13]

Perioperative BT results in better local control than surgery alone, though this benefit is limited to high-grade lesions. However, there are no data demonstrating the superiority or even equivalence of BT to EBRT.[15] A study from Fox Chase Cancer Center retrospectively compared the outcomes of patients treated with BT plus EBRT (25 patients) with those treated with EBRT alone (61 patients).[16] On univariate analysis, those treated with BT and EBRT had better local control at 5 years (100% vs 62%, $P = .03$), but no factors were significant on multivariate analysis.

ISOLATED LIMB PERFUSION

ILP uses the principle of local perfusion of high-dose chemotherapy (usually melphalan) and tumor necrosis factor α (TNF-α) under hyperthermic conditions. An oxygenated circuit is established by local arterial and venous cannulation on a bypass pump. A tourniquet is placed proximally, minimizing the risk of systemic circulation. ILP is widely available for melanoma, but few centers have significant experience with sarcoma.

Hyperthermic ILP may be considered in patients with locally advanced ESTS in whom a negative margin resection is unlikely or in individuals in whom local recurrence risks are high. ILP has been proved to shrink sarcomas, and is associated with high limb salvage rates and low local recurrence rates.[17–22] For instance, in a cohort of 55 patients with primary (30 patients) or recurrent (25 patients) unresectable ESTS, hyperthermic ILP with melphalan, interferon, and TNF-α permitted limb salvage in 84% secondary to a major response.[23]

However, no randomized controlled trials have compared ILP to alternative options, such as amputation or (neo)adjuvant therapy plus limb-sparing surgery. Thus, in reviewing the data that follows one must keep in mind that there are no data proving the superiority or even equivalence of this technique to more standard approaches.

ILP with chemotherapy alone is not as efficacious as ILP with chemotherapy plus TNF-α.[24] TNF-α has both an early and a late effect, enhancing tumor-selective uptake of melphalan or doxorubicin 3- to 6-fold during perfusion and, potentially, selective destruction of the tumor vasculature.[24] Higher doses of TNF-α do not seem to improve treatment efficacy but are associated with greater toxicity.[25]

A European multi-institutional trial enrolling 186 patients with locally advanced ESTS demonstrated that ILP with melphalan and TNF-α with or without interferon resulted in 18% clinical complete responses (CR) and 57% partial responses (PR). The limb salvage rate was 82%.[21] A single-institution retrospective study of 197 consecutive patients with limb-threatening ESTS undergoing 217 ILP procedures with melphalan and TNF-α at Erasmus MC-Daniel den Hoed Cancer Center demonstrated limb salvage rates of 87% with a perioperative mortality rate of 0.5%.[22] Multiple tumors and Stewart-Treves lymphangiosarcoma or Kaposi sarcoma were predictive of response on univariate analysis. Patients with stage IV disease undergoing ILP with palliative intent experienced overall response rates of 84% and limb salvage rates of 97%.

ILP followed by subsequent resection is associated with low local recurrence rates. In a retrospective review of 100 patients from a prospective database at Institut Gustave Roussy, hyperthermic ILP (38°–40°C) with melphalan (10 mg/L) and low-dose TNF-α (1 mg) followed by resection after 2 months was associated with a 79% response rate (CR and PR), 87% limb salvage rate, 89% 3-year OS rate, and 18% 3-year local recurrence rate.[19] Similarly, hyperthermic ILP with doxorubicin (instead of melphalan) and TNF-α in a series of 75 patients from the Italian Society of Integrated Locoregional Therapies in Oncology resulted in an 82% response rate, 85% limb-salvage rate, 63% 5-year locoregional DFS rate, 37% 5-year DFS rate, and 62% 5-year OS rate.[20]

A recent retrospective review of 122 patients with solitary locally advanced ESTS treated with melphalan and TNF-α ILP at Erasmus MC-Daniel den Hoed Cancer Center reported lower local recurrence rates in patients with R0 resections than in those with R1 resections (15% vs 28%, $P = .04$), and in those with greater than 50% ILP-induced tumor necrosis compared with those with 50% or less necrosis (7% vs 33%, $P = .001$).[26] None of the 36 patients with R0 resections and greater than 50% necrosis developed local recurrences, 21 of whom received no EBRT.

In experienced hands, this procedure is relatively well tolerated. Toxicity causing significant functional disturbances or threatened compartment syndrome (Wieberdink Acute Limb Toxicity Scale grade IV) or potentially requiring amputation (grade V) is rare,[19,22] and when noted is often observed with excessive muscular hyperthermia.[20] However, one series reported a 21% early complication rate (with 5% reoperation rate) and 23% long-term complication rate.[27] EBRT may be added as indicated, without increasing the burden of morbidity.[28]

ISOLATED LIMB INFUSION

More recently, ILI has been evaluated in the management of extremity sarcomas. Like ILP, ILI uses the same technique of circulating high-dose chemotherapy in an isolated extremity. In contrast, ILI is conducted through percutaneously placed catheters and is performed under hypoxic conditions.

There is limited experience with ILI in ESTS. In an Egyptian study of 40 patients with ESTS, ILI (with doxorubicin) and EBRT resulted in an 85% response rate and 83% limb-salvage rate.[29] The Sydney Melanoma Unit reported a 90% response rate and 62% DSS rate (median follow-up 28 months) to high-dose cytotoxic drug combination ILI in 21 patients with locally advanced ESTS.[30] Of interest, a lower initial skin temperature (median 35.8°C) was associated with a trend toward complete response ($P = .55$). A recent retrospective study of 14 ESTS from 5 institutions treated with melphalan/dactinomycin ILI demonstrated a 75% overall response rate (17% CR rate) and a 78% limb-salvage rate.[31] Median time to progression was 8.9 months.

Similar to ILP, ILI has not been directly compared with aggressive limb-sparing resection with EBRT in a randomized trial. It is arguable that patients under consideration for ILP and ILI are not necessarily candidates for surgery with EBRT at first evaluation. ILP and ILI should be considered as potential therapies in appropriately selected patients, and eligible patients should be referred to centers where this therapy is available.

CHEMOTHERAPY

Adjuvant and neoadjuvant chemotherapy remains controversial for the treatment of STS, except for rhabdomyosarcoma and Ewing sarcoma.[32] The Swedish Sarcoma Group randomized 240 patients with high-grade STS (86% extremity) between 1981 and 1986 to receive doxorubicin or no chemotherapy following radical surgery. Those with marginal resections additionally received postoperative RT. No significant differences in local control, DFS, or OS were observed at a median follow-up of 40 months.[33]

European Organization for the Research and Treatment of Cancer investigators reported pooled data from two phase III trials evaluating 819 patients with high-grade localized STS undergoing surgery treated with one of two adjuvant doxorubicin-based chemotherapy regimens (in one trial, cyclophosphamide, vincristine, doxorubicin, and dacarbazine [CYVADIC], and in the other, doxorubicin and ifosfamide [AI]).[34] The median follow-up was 8.2 years (CYVADIC trial, 468 patients, 9.7 years; AI trial, 351 patients, 6.6 years). Large-size, high-grade, and R1 resection were independent adverse prognostic factors for both progression-free survival (PFS) and OS. Those treated with chemotherapy demonstrated improved PFS but not OS. Males and patients older than 40 years had better PFS but not OS in the adjuvant chemotherapy arms. Chemotherapy was not associated with a better outcome in young patients. Patients who had undergone an R1 resection had better PFS and OS in the adjuvant chemotherapy arms. Therefore, the quality of the initial surgery was the most important prognostic and predictive factor associated with any potential benefit from adjuvant chemotherapy.

REGIONAL HYPERTHERMIA

The tumoricidal effects of temperature in excess of 40°C were demonstrated in 1967 in a rat hepatoma model, on a human melanoma cell line, and subsequently in humans.[35] Twenty-two patients (13 with sarcoma, 7 with melanoma, and 2 with squamous cell carcinoma) were treated with a 50-minute course of hyperthermic perfusate without chemotherapy using the ILP technique. There were 6 early deaths in the immediate postoperative period. Of the remaining 16 survivors, 12 were disease-free 3 to 28 months after treatment.[35]

As already described, hyperthermia has been combined with ILP. Most of the data regarding hyperthermia in sarcoma are in the context of ILP.

Regional hyperthermia is an entirely different concept, defined as controlled temperature elevation by targeting the heating field to the malignant tumor and the immediate surrounding tissue.[36] Hyperthermia is considered both a potent radiosensitizer and a potential chemosensitizer.[36] There are two principal treatment techniques for delivering hyperthermia. For superficial tumors, microwave-emitting applicators may be placed directly on the tumor surface. Deep-seated tumors may be treated with arrays of dipole antenna pairs arranged in a ring around the patient.

A phase III, multi-institutional trial randomized 341 patients with high-risk, deep STS at least 5 cm in size and classified as grade 2 or 3 by the Fédération Nationale des Centers de Lutte Contre le Cancer to receive neoadjuvant chemotherapy (etoposide, ifosfamide, and doxorubicin) with or without regional hyperthermia (169 and 172 patients, respectively).[37] Chemotherapy and hyperthermia were administered before and after surgery (91%) and radiation therapy (63%). Approximately 44% had ESTS. Hyperthermia was performed using an external radiofrequency source that achieved a tumoral temperature of 42°C. Response rates were higher with hyperthermia (29% vs 13%, $P = .002$). The 2-year local PFS was 76% for the hyperthermia group and 61% for the control group (relative hazard 0.58, 95% confidence interval [CI] 0.41–0.83; $P = .003$). For the subset with ESTS, local PFS rates of 92% versus 80% were not significantly different ($P = .2$). The cohort treated with hyperthermia experienced improved DFS ($P = .011$) and OS ($P = .038$). Combined therapy afforded

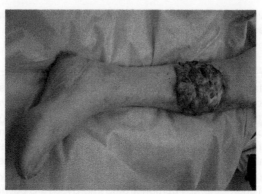

Fig. 6. Recurrent myxofibrosarcoma fungating through skin and associated with recurrent infections. Below-knee amputation was recommended.

a better OS with a hazard ratio of 0.88, without reaching significance. There were 3 deaths attributable to therapy, 2 in the hyperthermia group and 1 in the control group.[37]

While regional hyperthermia may increase the benefit of chemotherapy in some patients not adequately managed with surgery, large studies validating these results are necessary. Furthermore, significant benefit has not yet been demonstrated in patients with ESTS.

AMPUTATION

Limb salvage is generally possible even after local recurrences, and amputation should be considered as a last resort. After assessing all potential treatment and reconstructive options, it may impossible to salvage limb function. Amputation may be the only option, particularly in the case of a recurrent sarcoma encasing neurovascular structures when ILP/ILI and/or reconstruction are not feasible. A large fungating tumor may require resection or even amputation to reduce risk of hemorrhage or infection (**Fig. 6**). Furthermore, as previously mentioned, complications from recurrent tumor may necessitate amputation (see **Fig. 4**).

In a series of 413 patients with ESTS treated at the University of Toronto, 6% underwent amputation.[38] These patients were typically older ($P = .05$), had larger tumors ($P = .001$), and had greater risk of developing metastatic disease ($P = .008$) than those who underwent limb-sparing surgery. The main indication for a primary amputation of the upper extremity was severe functional compromise. Indications for amputation of the lower extremity included severe functional compromise, composite tissue involvement, and prior unplanned excision resulting in significant tissue contamination.

SUMMARY

Wide or radical limb-sparing, function-preserving surgery with negative margins is the standard of care for ESTS. RT reduces the risk of locoregional recurrence compared with surgery alone in many patients. Amputation is occasionally the only option (poor function, fungating tumor, fracture, field defect, neurovascular compromise), but given the similar OS rates after limb-sparing plus EBRT versus amputation, it should not be considered routinely. EBRT may be avoided if the risk of local recurrence is low, as with small tumors resected with wide margins. Recommendations may be tailored based on grade, depth, subsequent ability to salvage, and histology. BT is another local adjuvant radiation technique most beneficial in high-grade patients under certain circumstances. ILP/ILI may be offered to patients with locally advanced tumors with borderline resectability. The routine use of adjuvant and neoadjuvant chemotherapy outside of accepted and established protocols for certain histologies (such as Ewing sarcoma and rhabdomyosarcoma) remains controversial and is best offered in the context of a clinical trial. Regional hyperthermia at this time should be considered an experimental but potentially emerging technique that needs further validation.

REFERENCES

1. Lahat G, Lazar A, Lev D. Sarcoma epidemiology and etiology: potential environmental and genetic factors. Surg Clin North Am 2008;88:451–81, v.
2. Shiu MH, Castro EB, Hajdu SI, et al. Surgical treatment of 297 soft tissue sarcomas of the lower extremity. Ann Surg 1975;182:597–602.
3. Gronchi A, Lo Vullo S, Colombo C, et al. Extremity soft tissue sarcoma in a series of patients treated at a single institution: local control directly impacts survival. Ann Surg 2010;251:506–11.
4. Weitz J, Antonescu CR, Brennan MF. Localized extremity soft tissue sarcoma: improved knowledge with unchanged survival over time. J Clin Oncol 2003;21: 2719–25.
5. Gutierrez JC, Perez EA, Moffat FL, et al. Should soft tissue sarcomas be treated at high-volume centers? An analysis of 4205 patients. Ann Surg 2007;245:952–8.
6. Clark MA, Fisher C, Judson I, et al. Soft-tissue sarcomas in adults. N Engl J Med 2005;353:701–11.
7. Grimer R, Judson I, Peake D, et al. Guidelines for the management of soft tissue sarcomas. Sarcoma 2010;2010:506182.
8. Rosenberg SA, Tepper J, Glatstein E, et al. The treatment of soft-tissue sarcomas of the extremities: prospective randomized evaluations of (1) limb-sparing surgery plus radiation therapy compared with amputation and (2) the role of adjuvant chemotherapy. Ann Surg 1982;196:305–15.
9. Yang JC, Chang AE, Baker AR, et al. Randomized prospective study of the benefit of adjuvant radiation therapy in the treatment of soft tissue sarcomas of the extremity. J Clin Oncol 1998;16:197–203.
10. Baldini EH, Goldberg J, Jenner C, et al. Long-term outcomes after function-sparing surgery without radiotherapy for soft tissue sarcoma of the extremities and trunk. J Clin Oncol 1999;17:3252–9.
11. O'Sullivan B, Davis AM, Turcotte R, et al. Preoperative versus postoperative radiotherapy in soft-tissue sarcoma of the limbs: a randomised trial. Lancet 2002;359:2235–41.
12. Davis AM, O'Sullivan B, Turcotte R, et al. Late radiation morbidity following randomization to preoperative versus postoperative radiotherapy in extremity soft tissue sarcoma. Radiother Oncol 2005;75:48–53.
13. Brennan MF, Hilaris B, Shiu MH, et al. Local recurrence in adult soft-tissue sarcoma. A randomized trial of brachytherapy. Arch Surg 1987;122:1289–93.
14. Pisters PW, Harrison LB, Leung DH, et al. Long-term results of a prospective randomized trial of adjuvant brachytherapy in soft tissue sarcoma. J Clin Oncol 1996;14:859–68.
15. Raut CP, Albert M. Soft tissue sarcoma brachytherapy. In: Devlin PM, editor. Brachytherapy: applications and techniques. Philadelphia: Lippincott Williams & Wilkins; 2007. p. 269–310.

16. Andrews SF, Anderson PR, Eisenberg BL, et al. Soft tissue sarcomas treated with postoperative external beam radiotherapy with and without low-dose-rate brachytherapy. Int J Radiat Oncol Biol Phys 2004;59:475–80.

17. Eggermont AM, de Wilt JH, ten Hagen TL. Current uses of isolated limb perfusion in the clinic and a model system for new strategies. Lancet Oncol 2003;4: 429–37.

18. Hayes AJ, Neuhaus SJ, Clark MA, et al. Isolated limb perfusion with melphalan and tumor necrosis factor alpha for advanced melanoma and soft-tissue sarcoma. Ann Surg Oncol 2007;14:230–8.

19. Bonvalot S, Rimareix F, Causeret S, et al. Hyperthermic isolated limb perfusion in locally advanced soft tissue sarcoma and progressive desmoid-type fibromatosis with TNF 1 mg and melphalan (T1-M HILP) is safe and efficient. Ann Surg Oncol 2009;16:3350–7.

20. Di Filippo F, Giacomini P, Rossi CR, et al. Hyperthermic isolated perfusion with tumor necrosis factor-alpha and doxorubicin for the treatment of limb-threatening soft tissue sarcoma: the experience of the Italian Society of Integrated Locoregional Treatment in Oncology (SITILO). In Vivo 2009;23:363–7.

21. Eggermont AM, Schraffordt Koops H, Klausner JM, et al. Isolated limb perfusion with tumor necrosis factor and melphalan for limb salvage in 186 patients with locally advanced soft tissue extremity sarcomas. The cumulative multicenter European experience. Ann Surg 1996;224:756–64 [discussion: 64–5].

22. Grunhagen DJ, de Wilt JH, Graveland WJ, et al. Outcome and prognostic factor analysis of 217 consecutive isolated limb perfusions with tumor necrosis factor-alpha and melphalan for limb-threatening soft tissue sarcoma. Cancer 2006; 106:1776–84.

23. Eggermont AM, Schraffordt Koops H, Lienard D, et al. Isolated limb perfusion with high-dose tumor necrosis factor-alpha in combination with interferon-gamma and melphalan for nonresectable extremity soft tissue sarcomas: a multicenter trial. J Clin Oncol 1996;14:2653–65.

24. Verhoef C, de Wilt JH, Grunhagen DJ, et al. Isolated limb perfusion with melphalan and TNF-alpha in the treatment of extremity sarcoma. Curr Treat Options Oncol 2007;8:417–27.

25. Bonvalot S, Laplanche A, Lejeune F, et al. Limb salvage with isolated perfusion for soft tissue sarcoma: could less TNF-alpha be better? Ann Oncol 2005;16:1061–8.

26. Deroose JP, Burger JW, van Geel AN, et al. Radiotherapy for soft tissue sarcomas after isolated limb perfusion and surgical resection: essential for local control in all patients? Ann Surg Oncol 2011;18:321–7.

27. Cherix S, Speiser M, Matter M, et al. Isolated limb perfusion with tumor necrosis factor and melphalan for non-resectable soft tissue sarcomas: long-term results on efficacy and limb salvage in a selected group of patients. J Surg Oncol 2008;98:148–55.

28. Olieman AF, Pras E, van Ginkel RJ, et al. Feasibility and efficacy of external beam radiotherapy after hyperthermic isolated limb perfusion with TNF-alpha and melphalan for limb-saving treatment in locally advanced extremity soft-tissue sarcoma. Int J Radiat Oncol Biol Phys 1998;40:807–14.

29. Hegazy MA, Kotb SZ, Sakr H, et al. Preoperative isolated limb infusion of doxorubicin and external irradiation for limb-threatening soft tissue sarcomas. Ann Surg Oncol 2007;14:568–76.

30. Moncrieff MD, Kroon HM, Kam PC, et al. Isolated limb infusion for advanced soft tissue sarcoma of the extremity. Ann Surg Oncol 2008;15:2749–56.

31. Turaga KK, Beasley GM, Kane JM 3rd, et al. Limb preservation with isolated limb infusion for locally advanced nonmelanoma cutaneous and soft-tissue malignant neoplasms. Arch Surg 2011;146:870–5.

32. Bacci G, Picci P, Gitelis S, et al. The treatment of localized Ewing's sarcoma: the experience at the Istituto Ortopedico Rizzoli in 163 cases treated with and without adjuvant chemotherapy. Cancer 1982;49:1561–70.

33. Alvegard TA, Sigurdsson H, Mouridsen H, et al. Adjuvant chemotherapy with doxorubicin in high-grade soft tissue sarcoma: a randomized trial of the Scandinavian Sarcoma Group. J Clin Oncol 1989;7:1504–13.

34. Le Cesne A, Woll PJ, Bramwell VH, et al. The end of adjuvant chemotherapy (adCT) era with doxorubicin-based regimen in resected high-grade soft tissue sarcoma (STS): pooled analysis of the two STBSG-EORTC phase III clinical trials. J Clin Oncol 2008;26:10525.

35. Cavaliere R, Ciocatto EC, Giovanella BC, et al. Selective heat sensitivity of cancer cells. Biochemical and clinical studies. Cancer 1967;20:1351–81.

36. Lindner LH, Issels RD. Hyperthermia in soft tissue sarcoma. Curr Treat Options Oncol 2011;12:12–20.

37. Issels RD, Lindner LH, Verweij J, et al. Neo-adjuvant chemotherapy alone or with regional hyperthermia for localised high-risk soft-tissue sarcoma: a randomised phase 3 multicentre study. Lancet Oncol 2010;11:561–70.

38. Ghert MA, Abudu A, Driver N, et al. The indications for and the prognostic significance of amputation as the primary surgical procedure for localized soft tissue sarcoma of the extremity. Ann Surg Oncol 2005;12:10–7.

Radiation Therapy: Neoadjuvant, Adjuvant, or Not at All

Thomas F. DeLaney, MD[a,b,*]

KEYWORDS

- Soft tissue sarcoma • Radiation therapy • Adjuvant
- Neoadjuvant

OVERVIEW

The major therapeutic goals in the treatment of soft tissue sarcomas (STSs) are survival and local tumor control (LC) with the lowest achievable morbidity. For extremity lesions, another important goal is optimal limb function. Surgical resection of the primary tumor is an essential component of treatment for virtually all patients (although not discussed in detail in this article, radiation therapy [RT] alone can be an effective treatment for selected patients who are medically inoperable or who decline surgery).[1] A high-quality surgical margin is necessary for LC when surgery is used without radiation (ie, the surgical plane of dissection should traverse normal tissue outside the reactive tumor zone).[2] This is because STSs tend to infiltrate normal tissue adjacent to the evident lesion.[3] Thus, removal of the gross lesion by a simple excision alone (only a narrow margin) is followed by high rates of local recurrence (LR).[4] Radical resections are associated with a reduction in the LR rate but, in cases of extremity STS, may compromise limb function. For retroperitoneal tumors, they may still fail to achieve LC because of the many adjacent critical structures that cannot be excised. The combination of conservative surgery and RT has been shown in randomized controlled studies to achieve higher rates of LC than surgery alone.[5,6] Selected patients, generally those with superficial T1 ($\leq$5 cm) lesions that can be widely excised with acceptable margins, can be well managed by surgery alone without RT.[2] Good limb function is achieved in the majority of patients with extremity sarcomas; acute[7] and late[8] RT-associated morbidity are seen in some patients undergoing RT. One focus of current STS clinical

Disclosures: The author has nothing to disclose.
[a] Harvard Medical School, Boston, MA, USA
[b] Department of Radiation Oncology, Francis H. Burr Proton Therapy Center, Center for Sarcoma and Connective Tissue Oncology, Massachusetts General Hospital, 55 Fruit Street, Boston, MA 02114, USA
* Department of Radiation Oncology, Francis H. Burr Proton Therapy Center, Center for Sarcoma and Connective Tissue Oncology, Massachusetts General Hospital, 55 Fruit Street, Boston, MA 02114.
E-mail address: tdelaney@partners.org

trials is the evaluation of techniques and technologies to potentially reduce the risk of radiation-associated morbidity;[9,10] details of Radiation Therapy Oncology Group clinical studies looking at these questions can be accessed at the following website (http://www.rtog.org/ClinicalTrials/ProtocolTable/StudyDetails.aspx?study=0630), data from these studies are emerging and are discussed later. There are no published randomized studies of which the author is aware that compare surgery alone with surgery and adjuvant RT for retroperitoneal STS. Nevertheless there are data to suggest that radiation can enhance LC for the retroperitoneal tumors with acceptable morbidity when sophisticated radiation techniques are combined with radical resections performed by experienced oncologic surgeons with expertise in managing sarcomas.[11] Advances in RT in this area are discussed.

Because both surgical and radiation techniques are critical for optimizing LC of tumor and functional outcome with acceptable morbidity, it is important to manage these patients in dedicated multispecialty centers composed of physicians with expertise in STS, including orthopedic oncologists, surgical oncologists, plastic surgeons, radiation oncologists, medical oncologists, sarcoma pathologists, and bone and soft tissue diagnostic radiologists.[12] RT may involve external beam RT, which can be 3-D conformal or intensity-modulated RT (IMRT), and use photons or protons, brachytherapy (BRT), intraoperative RT, or combinations thereof. External beam RT can be given either preoperatively or postoperatively. The clinical considerations and the outcome data that must be considered in choosing the most appropriate treatment technique for individual patients are discussed. Although there are similar general considerations for extremity, truncal, head and neck, and retroperitoneal sarcomas, there are sufficient differences in behavior, as well as in surgical and radiation techniques and their underlying rationale, that this discussion is divided into separate sections on extremity/truncal and retroperitoneal sarcomas. In the interest of time and space, the role of adjuvant RT in the management of head/neck and gynecologic or visceral sarcomas and the use of RT in the management of pediatric rhabdomyosarcoma are not discussed. Although the clinical behavior of the pediatric nonrhabdomyosarcoma STSs seems similar to that of the adult STSs, management considerations related to growth retardation and other potential toxicities of RT that are particularly relevant to pediatric patients are sufficiently different that the use of adjuvant RT for these tumors also are not addressed.

EXTREMITY AND TRUNCAL STS
Introduction

Because STSs tend to infiltrate normal tissue adjacent to the tumor, simple excision alone is followed by LR in 60% to 90% of patients.[4] Radical resection of a wider margin of apparently normal tissue around the tumor reduces the LR rate to approximately 25% to 30%.[13] With the use of compartmental resections, the LR rate drops to 10% to 20% with surgery alone.[13] One study that reported a zero LR rate derives from the amputation arm of the National Cancer Institute trial comparing amputation with limb salvage treatment.[14] Careful selection of patients and attention to technique in some recent series, however, has achieved high rates of LC in selected patients (generally with smaller, lower-grade lesions) with conservative surgery alone.[2,15]

For the majority of patients with extremity STS undergoing conservative surgery, RT is also used to achieve a high rate of LC with good functional result.[7,14,16,17] The rationale for combining RT with surgery is to avoid the functional and cosmetic deformity associated with radical resection and to avoid the late consequences of high RT doses to large volumes of normal tissue in patients treated with primary RT alone. RT at moderate-dose levels (50–65 Gy) is as effective as radical resection in eradicating the microscopic extensions beyond the gross lesion, resulting in similar high rates of LC.[14] This has allowed maximization of functional and cancer-related outcome without the significant morbidity of radical surgery. Most centers report LC rates of approximately 90% with the combination of margin-negative limb-sparing surgery and RT for high-grade extremity STSs and 90% to 100% for low-grade STSs depending on the size.[14,18–25]

In addition to its benefit in improving LC rates, adjunctive RT has had a significant impact on limb salvage for extremity STSs. As an example, in the 1970s, 50% of patients with extremity STS underwent amputation; those patients treated by wide excision alone with limb preservation experienced a 30% rate of LR. With the subsequent application of RT and advanced reconstructive techniques, the rate of primary amputation at major centers has been reduced to approximately 5%, and the incidence of LR with limb preservation has been reduced to 10% to 15% without any measurable decrease in overall survival (OS).[14,26–28] A single, prospective randomized trial showed similar rates of disease-free survival and OS for patients treated with amputation or the combination of limb-sparing surgery and RT for extremity STS.[14]

Selection of Patients for Surgical Resection Alone (No RT)

Because of potential acute and late morbidity from RT, it is important to select patients who may be effectively treated with surgery alone. Several published series have evaluated wide-excision limb-sparing surgery alone. In one report, 119 selected patients with extremity STS were grouped according to anatomic location as subcutaneous (n = 40), intramuscular (n = 30), or extramuscular (n = 49).[29] The 70 patients with subcutaneous and intramuscular tumors were all treated by local surgery, and a wide margin (requiring a cuff of fat tissue around the tumor and inclusion of the deep fascia beneath the tumor) was obtained in 56. These patients were followed without postoperative RT. During a median follow-up of 5 years (range, 3.5–10 years), only 4 had an LR, despite 84% having had high-grade tumors. The investigators concluded that postoperative RT may not be necessary in this subgroup. A similar study at the MD Anderson Cancer Center evaluated LC for T1 tumors after excision alone with negative margins. Wide local excision was performed with the intent of including a 1-cm to 2-cm margin of normal tissue around the mass. Negative surgical margins were achieved in 84% of the 88 enrolled patients; the remaining 16% with microscopically positive margins received postoperative RT. In those with excision alone, the 5-year LR rate was 7.9%, and the 5-year sarcoma-specific death rate was 3.2%.[30] In another study, 74 patients with localized STS of the extremity or trunk underwent function-sparing surgery without RT.[2] The overall 10-year actuarial LC rate was 93% and was dependent on the adequacy of surgical margins (87% for patients with margins of less than 1 cm versus 100% for patients with margins of 1 cm or more). The 10-year survival rate was 73%. This approach may be appropriate for carefully selected patients with small (<5 cm) superficial tumors or small deep tumors that can be resected with all margins greater than or equal to 1 cm (or perhaps less if an intervening fascial barrier).

Surgical Resection Combined with RT

The recommended treatment for most patients who are medically and technically operable is the combination of function-preserving surgery and RT, with the exception of the minority of patients with small, generally superficial lesions that can be widely excised with negative margins and good functional results. In most instances, the probability of LC and the late functional and cosmetic results are superior using this combined modality approach. RT is an effective treatment of STS because the radiation sensitivity of cell lines derived from sarcomas is not less than that of epithelial cell lines.[31] For small sarcomas, good LC rates can be achieved by RT alone. LC probabilities of more than 90% for tumors of estimated volumes of 15 mL to 65 mL (approximately a sphere of 3–5 cm in diameter), however, require high radiation doses (>75 Gy).[32] For unresected sarcomas, there seems to be an advantage for doses above 63 Gy.[1] Because most treatment volumes are large, the late normal tissue changes resulting from these dose levels are clinically important in nearly all patients. In animal models, a significantly lower radiation dose is required to achieve LC when RT is combined with simple excision than with RT alone.[33]

The impact of combined modality treatment that includes external beam RT on both LC and survival has been evaluated in only one prospective randomized trial. In this study, 91 patients with high-grade lesions were randomly assigned to surgery plus postoperative chemotherapy with or without postoperative adjuvant external beam RT, and 50 with low-grade lesions were randomized to surgery plus adjuvant external beam RT or surgery alone.[6] In the patients with high-grade lesions, there were no LRs in the patients randomized to external beam RT, whereas the patients receiving only adjuvant chemotherapy had a 22% actuarial LR rate at 10 years. In patients with low-grade sarcoma, the LR rates were 4% versus 33% in the postoperative RT and surgery alone groups, respectively. There was no influence of postoperative RT on OS for either high-grade or low-grade tumors.

Preoperative (Neoadjuvant) Versus Postoperative (Adjuvant) RT

There are potential advantages to both preoperative and postoperative administration of RT. Preoperative RT might reduce tumor burden before resection, theoretically allowing more conservative surgical therapy. RT fields can be limited to the tumor and adjacent tissues at risk for microscopic infiltration, a volume that is considerably smaller than that which must be treated after surgery, where the entire surgical bed is included in the initial target volume irradiated to 50 Gy. RT doses are lower (50 Gy preoperative vs 60–66 Gy postoperative). Postoperative RT allows histologic examination of a tumor specimen, especially the margins, aiding in further treatment planning; it is also associated with fewer acute wound complications.

There is one randomized controlled study comparing preoperative with postoperative RT. This study was designed to evaluate the incidence of acute wound healing complications in patients with potentially curable extremity STS.[34] In this Canadian trial, 190 patients were randomly assigned to either preoperatively RT (50 Gy preoperatively for all 94 patients randomized to this arm with 16–20 Gy postoperative boost reserved for the 14 patients in this arm with a positive margin) or postoperative RT (50 Gy initial field + 16–20 Gy boost field for all patients). Complications were defined as secondary wound surgery, hospital admission for wound care, or the need for deep packing or prolonged wound dressings within 120 days of tumor resection.

The study was terminated when a highly significant result was obtained at the time of a planned interim analysis. With a median follow-up of 3.3 years, a significantly higher percentage of preoperatively treated patients had acute wound complications (35% vs 17%). Other factors associated with wound complications were the volume of resected tissue and lower limb location of the tumor. Late morbidity was initially not reported. Because the RT fields for the postoperative RT were larger and the dose delivered for most patients was higher, the investigators indicated that more follow-up would be needed to assess whether these larger RT volumes and higher RT doses would lead to more late treatment effects in these patients.

In a later publication, the LR rate, regional or distant failure rate, progression-free survival, and functional outcome did not differ between the groups.[35] These data have been updated with a median follow-up of 6.9 years. There remain no differences in LC between the patients in the 2 arms of the study with more than 90% LC. The regional and distant failure rates as well as the progression-free and OS rates are also no different between the 2 arms of the study.[36] The postoperative RT patients, however, have greater 5-year actuarial rates of grade 2 to grade 4 late toxicity (86%) when compared with the preoperative patients (68%) (P = .0002). Subcutaneous toxicity rated as grade 3 (severe induration and loss of subcutaneous tissue or field contracture greater than 10% linear measurement) or grade 4 (necrosis) was significantly more common in the postoperative group, 36% versus 23% (P = .02).

There is, thus, a difference in the morbidity profile between preoperative RT and postoperative RT. A higher rate of generally reversible acute wound healing complications occurred in patients receiving preoperative treatment, which was offset by a higher rate of generally irreversible late complications, including grades 3 and 4 fibrosis, in patients receiving postoperative RT. Because few acute wound healing complications occurred in either group when the tumor was in the upper extremity, it seems prudent to treat these patients with preoperative RT. The author has also favored preoperative RT for the majority of patients with lower extremity tumors, because acute wound complications can usually be managed and go on to heal whereas the late treatment effects are usually permanent. For patients with lower extremity lesions, this study makes it clear that new strategies are needed to (1) reduce the risk of acute wound healing problems when patients receive preoperative RT and (2) reduce the risk of late treatment–induced effects when higher-dose, larger-field postoperative RT is given.

Brachytherapy

Compared with external beam RT, BRT minimizes the radiation dose to surrounding normal tissues, maximizes the RT dose delivered to the tumor, and shortens treatment times. In the usual dosage schedule, treatment is completed within 5 days and requires only one hospitalization. At the time of surgery, afterloading catheters are placed in a target area of the tumor operative bed, defined by the surgeon, and spaced at 1-cm intervals to cover the entire area of risk (**Fig. 1**). BRT can also be used for delivery of a boost to the tumor bed in conjunction with external beam RT.[37]

A phase III trial of postoperative BRT versus no BRT was conducted in 126 patients who had complete resection of either extremity STS or superficial trunk STS.[22] The BRT dose was 45 Gy using low dose rate iridium Ir 192. The 5-year LC rates were 82% and 67% for the BRT and surgery alone groups, respectively. The advantage of BRT was seen only in the high-grade sarcomas[5,22] and was limited to LC, because there was no difference between the groups in distant metastasis or disease-specific survival.[22]

Although it is unclear whether BRT is associated with a higher risk of wound complications (discussed later), the rate of wound reoperation may be higher.[38] BRT has been combined with free flap construction as a means of enhancing primary healing in difficult anatomic situations without an increase in the incidence of wound breakdown.[39] There have been no randomized comparisons of the relative efficacy or morbidity of external beam RT with BRT.

The Memorial Sloan-Kettering Cancer Center group recently did a retrospective comparison of patients who had received adjuvant RT with IMRT (discussed later) to a group of patients who had received adjuvant brachytherapy.[40] A higher rate of LC was noted in the IMRT group in spite of higher risk features in that group. On

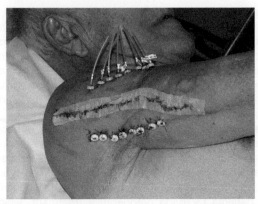

Fig. 1. High-dose BRT catheters in place in an 83-year-old man with a history of a prior grade 3/3 malignant fibrous histiocytoma of the soft tissues of his right arm excised originally in 1992 followed by postoperative adjuvant RT, who has now undergone excision and BRT treatment of what was either LR tumor or a radiation-associated second tumor 18 years later.

the basis of this analysis, they have adopted IMRT as their standard adjuvant RT technique. They did not compare IMRT with 3-D conformal RT. Because the RT treatment target volumes are similar between IMRT and 3-D conformal RT, a difference in LC with these 2 external beam techniques was not expected, although morbidity may differ.

BRT for sarcomas has traditionally been given by low dose rate. There are emerging data on the use of fractionated high dose rate schedules.[41–43] High dose rate BRT has been used in conjunction with external beam RT for the tumor bed boost in doses of 15 Gy to 24 Gy, often hyperfractionated at 2.3 Gy to 4 Gy twice a day.[42] Early retrospective evidence suggests that comparable rates of LC can be achieved when combining either low dose rate or high dose rate BT with external beam RT.[44] One report using high dose rate BRT alone in doses of 40 Gy at 2.3 Gy to 3 Gy twice a day, however, reported poor LC of only 20% in contrast to 100% when BRT was combined with external beam RT.[43]

External Beam RT Treatment Planning

The RT treatment technique should be carefully planned so that the tissues irradiated are only those judged at risk. To use the smallest target volumes, the part to be irradiated must be securely and reproducibly immobilized, which generally involves customized immobilization, typically with moldable thermoplastic (**Fig. 2**). Treatment is planned by performing a CT scan of the immobilized, affected extremity. This is facilitated by the availability of a large bore scanner that allows maximum flexibility in arranging the limb such that the contralateral extremity and the trunk will be out the treatment beams. Treatment planning is enhanced by the ability to fuse the RT planning CT scan with the MRI scan. A radiation oncologist defines the target volumes (on each section of the CT/MRI of the affected region); target definition may be improved by review of the planning studies jointly by the radiation oncologist, surgeon, and diagnostic radiologist. The radiation oncologist also defines nontarget critical structures in the treatment volume, specifies dose constraints for these, and then works with the dosimetrists to design treatment techniques that achieve the closest feasible conformation of treatment to target volumes (**Fig. 3**). This may require

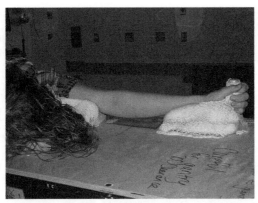

Fig. 2. Customized immobilization device for a patient with a synovial sarcoma of the soft tissues of the left forearm, incompletely excised via a transverse incision by a surgeon who thought this might be a benign lesion. The patient is receiving preoperative radiation before tumor bed re-excision.

complex field arrangements, treatment angles, gapped fields, wedge filters, tissue compensators, bolus, and/or intensity modulation. In general, the radiation oncologist attempts to:

- Avoid inclusion of an entire joint space.
- Avoid full-dose RT of adjacent bone to reduce the risk of pathologic fracture.
- Use wedges and tissue compensators as needed to account for tissue heterogeneities and minimize dose inhomogeneity.
- Incorporate an appropriate planning target volume expansion to account for treatment setup variability and any target motion.
- Review the treatment plan at multiple levels along the extremity to assess dose homogeneity to the target and normal tissues.

RT Treatment Volumes and Dose

The extent of normal tissue to be irradiated adjacent to the tumor bed in cases of preoperative RT and adjacent to the surgical bed in cases of postoperative RT is not definitively known. Few patterns of failure studies that relate the extent of the RT field to the site of LR have been reported. Because sarcomas are judged to infiltrate along rather than through tissue planes, longitudinal margins proximally and distally have traditionally been considerably more generous than radial margins. Historically, fields that extended from the muscle origin to insertion[45] or provided generous proximal/distal margins on the tumor were used.[46] In some centers from the 1970s through the mid-1990s, 5-cm to 10-cm proximal and distal block margins were used for large grade 1 and small grade 2 lesions and more generous fields with 10-cm to 15-cm margins encompassed large grade 2 to grade 3 lesions.[46] The advent of improved MRI delineation of tumor extent and subsequent surgical experience showing high rates of LC with surgical margins greater than or equal to 1 cm or including fascial barriers prompted radiation oncologists to use proximal/distal margins of 5 cm or less for small grade 1 lesions and 5-cm to 7-cm proximal/distal margins for larger, higher-grade lesions. Newer (3-D) treatment planning systems seem to allow smaller and more accurate treatment volumes in patients with extremity STS.

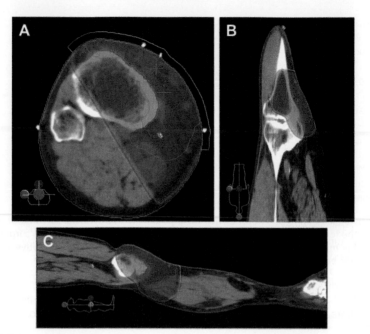

Fig. 3. A 3-D conformal RT plan—(A) axial, (B) coronal, and (C) sagittal—for a 76-year-old man who had undergone an unplanned excision of a grade 2-3/3 epithelioid myxofibrosarcoma of the soft tissues overlying the medial aspect of the left tibia, now receiving 50 Gy in 25 fractions via left anterior and right posterior oblique 6-MV photon fields. (*Courtesy of Brian Napolitano, BS, CMD, Massachusetts General Hospital, Boston, MA.*)

There are few studies in the literature looking at the appropriate target volume used when planning RT for extremity STS. One group found a remarkable difference in 5-year LC where the margin was less than 5 cm (30%) or at least 5 cm (93%).[47] These data conflict with the BRT data, where acceptable results are achieved using margins 2-cm longitudinally and 1.5 cm to 2 cm laterally. A study from the Royal Marsden hospital has suggested that, as in other tumor sites, the great majority of LRs occur within the high-dose volume.[48] The use of 5-cm proximal and distal block margins and 2-cm radial block margins (on the tumor for preoperative RT or on the surgical bed for postoperative RT) for the first 50 Gy provided high rates of LC in the randomized National Cancer Institute of Canada trial (discussed previously).[7]

A recent retrospective study lends valuable insight into optimal field size in preoperative RT. Patterns of LR were evaluated in 56 patients who underwent preoperative RT to a median dose of 50 Gy. The field size used for all patients was a clinical target volume (CTV) that included the T1 postgadolinium tumor with a 1-cm to 1.5-cm radial margin and 3.5-cm longitudinal margin, with an additional expansion of 5 mm to 7 mm to define the planning target volume. Boost doses of 10 Gy to 20 Gy were administered to the 12 patients with close or positive margins. The 5-year actuarial LC rate of 88.5% was comparable to other series. Tumor size and surgical margin status were the primary predictors of LR. All 5 LRs occurred in patients with either positive resection margins or resection margins of less than 1 mm. No LRs occurred in those with margins of 1 mm or greater. Although good LC rates were achieved, all LRs occurred within the preoperative CTV.[49] The target volume issue is complicated by the variety of histologic subtypes of STS, including some with a very infiltrative biology, such as myxofibrosarcoma,[50] which may require wider fields than some other more circumscribed tumors.

This study raises questions as to whether the more traditional large-volume primary RT field is necessary and whether the boost is necessary when an adequate surgical margin has been achieved. These questions are particularly relevant because of the advent of techniques, such as IMRT and protons, that can allow selective sparing of normal tissues. It is important to determine the volumes that can safely be spared before these techniques can be optimally implemented. Such studies are currently being conducted by cooperative groups in the United States and Europe. A phase II study by the Radiation Therapy Oncology Group (RTOG), which completed accrual in September 2010, is evaluating the role of image-guided RT (cone beam CT, tomotherapy, and so forth) in delivering preoperative RT to patients with extremity STS using more limited CTV margins (RTOG study 0630). CTVs in this study encompass the T1 postgadolinium enhancing region plus a 3-cm longitudinal margin and 1.5-cm radial margin for intermediate-grade or high-grade tumors that are 8 cm or greater. For all other tumors, a 2-cm longitudinal margin and a 1-cm radial margin are used. The primary outcome of interest is toxicity 2 years after treatment, and secondary outcomes will evaluate LC and other survival measures.

Another study, performed by investigators in Toronto, that needs to be carefully considered in the discussion of RT volumes, correlates MRI and surgical findings in patients undergoing surgery without any neoadjuvant therapy. It provided a histologic assessment of peritumoral edema as demonstrated by increased T2-weighted signal intensity on MRI scans performed preoperatively on 15 patients with high-grade extremity or truncal sarcomas ranging from 3.1 cm to 30.1 cm (mean 13.8 cm).[3] The extent of peritumoral T2-weighted signal intensity changes beyond the tumor ranged from 0 cm to 7.1 cm (mean 2.5 cm); contrast enhancement ranged from 0 cm to 5.3 cm (mean 1.1 cm). Tumor cells were identified histologically in the tissues beyond the gross tumor in 10 of 15 cases. In 6 cases, the tumor cells were located within 1 cm of the tumor margin, and in 4 cases, malignant cells were found at a distance greater than 1 cm and up to 4 cm. The location of the tumor cells did not correlate with tumor size or extent of peritumoral changes on the MRI scans. In 9 of 10 cases, however, the tumor cells were identified histologically in areas with corresponding high T2-weighted signal changes on MRI. With ever-increasing ability of the available RT technology to conform the RT dose to the target, this study has significant implications for RT target design and must be considered in future studies of RT volumes in this disease.

The radial CTV margins should be viewed with respect to the direction of most likely spread and are rationally derived from surgical series with high rates of LC without adjuvant RT with surgical margins greater than or equal to 1 cm or an intervening fascial barrier. Because the gross tumor delineation with RT planning imaging is less precise than that achievable in the operating room, radial CTV margins of 1.5 cm to 2.0 cm with approximately 0.5 cm for planning target volume expansion are added to account for daily setup variation. Where there is intervening bone, interosseous membrane, or major fascial planes and these planes are intact in the imaging studies, the radial CTV margins can be constricted to the surface of these structures. When a fascial plane has been violated, wider margins are appropriate to cover areas of potential contamination by tumor.

For patients receiving preoperative RT, 50 Gy is administered over 5 weeks, followed 3 to 5 weeks later by a conservative resection. For patients with negative surgical margins and no other unfavorable prognostic features, such as tumor cutthrough or satellite lesions after prior surgical interventions, 50 Gy of preoperative

RT seems sufficient to provide LC in a high proportion of patients. Sadoski and colleagues[51] analyzed 132 consecutive patients with STS of the extremities treated with preoperative RT and resectional surgery and found that (1) the 5-year actuarial LC rates were 97% and 81% for patients with negative margins and positive margins, respectively (this difference was highly significant); (2) there was no difference in LC between the various subcategories of negative margins (negative at <1 mm, 96%; negative at greater than 1 mm, 97%; not measured, 94%; and no tumor in the specimen, 100%); (3) there was no difference in LC for treatment of primary and LR lesions (after previous surgery alone) when the tumors were stratified for margin status; and (4) for the patients with negative margin, LC was not a function of STS size.

For patients with positive margins after preoperative RT, it has generally been recommended to use a shrinking treatment volume technique with delivery of either BRT or a postoperative external beam RT boost dose of 16 Gy to 18 Gy to the tumor bed once the surgical wound has healed. A boost dose to 66 Gy is given postoperatively or intraoperatively for microscopically positive margins and to 75 Gy if there is gross residual disease. In patients with frozen section evidence of close or positive margins, a boost dose can be administered intraoperatively using BRT or electron beam. For BRT, it is appropriate to deliver approximately 16 Gy by low dose rate techniques or 14 Gy to 16 Gy by high dose rate given as 3.5 Gy to 4 Gy twice a day for microscopically positive margins. Gross residual disease needs a dose of approximately 20 Gy to 25 Gy. Although delivery of a postoperative RT boost after resection with positive margins remains the standard of care, its efficacy in achieving LC has been called into question by the results of at least one retrospective study using external beam RT.[52]

For patients undergoing postoperative RT, irradiation usually begins 14 to 20 days after surgery, once the wound is healed. After resection of large tumors, it may be necessary to wait 3 to 4 weeks to allow resorption of the seroma. The initial volume must include all tissues handled during the surgical procedure, including the drain site, often encompassing the surgical bed with an initial CTV of approximately 4 cm proximally and distally and 1.5 to 2 cm radially. The dose to the initial CTV is 50 Gy. Progressively shrinking treatment volumes are then used to encompass the tumor bed and, if needed, areas of positive margins or gross residual disease; the final dose is 60 Gy for volumes with negative margins, 66 to 68 Gy for areas of positive margins or LR disease,[53] and 75 Gy for gross residual sarcoma.

The available information on a dose-response relationship for LC of extremity STS treated with surgery and postoperative RT is somewhat conflicting. Mundt and colleagues[47] reported that LC was dose dependent. Although postoperative patients receiving less than 60 Gy had worse LC than those receiving 60 Gy or more, no difference was seen in LC between patients receiving 60 Gy to 63.9 Gy (74.4%) and those receiving 64 Gy to 66 Gy (87.0%) ($P = .5$). Severe late sequelae were more frequent in patients treated with doses of 63 Gy or more than in patients treated with lower doses (23.1% vs 0%).[47]

Fein and colleagues[54] reported that patients receiving less than 62.5 Gy had a 5-year LC of 78% versus 95% in those with a dose greater than 62.5 Gy. In a multivariate analysis of patients undergoing postoperative RT, Zagars and Ballo[53] identified dose as an independent variable for LC. Doses of 64 Gy or more correlated with improved LC. Recognizing that the effectiveness of a particular dose was also related to other factors influencing LC, such as margin status, anatomic site, and LR presentation, they recommended postoperative doses of 60 Gy for patients with negative margins and otherwise favorable prognostic features while suggesting increasing doses for less favorable presentations, up to doses of 68 Gy for positive margins. In contrast, other investigators have not been able to demonstrate a clear dose-response relationship in reviews of their patients undergoing postoperative RT.[27,55-57] In practice, most centers give 60 Gy of postoperative RT for patients with negative margins and 66 Gy to 68 Gy for positive margins, using shrinking fields (described previously).

With regard to preoperative RT, Robinson and colleagues[58] failed to demonstrate a variation in LC according to dose, although the response rate to preoperative RT was clearly dose dependent. The accepted dose for preoperative RT is 50 Gy.

For treatment of an extremity STS, a good functional result demands that a portion of the cross-section of the extremity be spared from high-dose RT.[59] Thus, some tissue should not be irradiated to high dose to avoid compromising lymphatic drainage. For large tumors that are treated with wide resection, there may be persistent leg edema, requiring the use of a pressure-type stocking, even though the RT treatment volume is less than circumferential. This may be a problem for patients with large (>10 cm) sarcomas of the medial thigh.

When postoperative RT is combined with adjuvant chemotherapy, RT daily dose has been reduced in some series by 10% from 200 cGy to 180 cGy; RT is not given concurrently with doxorubicin. Instead, 2 to 3 days are allowed between the doxorubicin and RT. Some preoperative protocols have interdigitated chemotherapy and RT (discussed later); total preoperative RT has been reduced (ie, 44 Gy) in this setting.

Intensity-Modulated Photon RT

The purpose of RT is to maximize the dose delivered to the tumor while minimizing the exposure of dose-sensitive critical structures to high dose. This has been achieved traditionally by shaping the spatial distribution of the high RT dose to conform to the target volume (hence, 3-D conformal RT), thereby reducing the dose to the nontarget structures. Although this approach is satisfactory in the treatment of targets that are approximately convex in shape, it is less than optimal for targets that contain complex concavities or that wrap around critical structures.[60] Growing experience suggests that IMRT plans produce dose distributions for patients that are superior to 3-D conformal plans, both in terms of dose conformity around the tumor and dose reduction to the specified critical normal structures, albeit at the cost of irradiating a larger volume of normal tissue with a low to moderate dose (**Fig. 4**). Dosimetric studies comparing IMRT with conformal RT for STS have been reported. When evaluating sarcomas arising in the extremities, pelvis, trunk, and paranasal sinuses, IMRT plans were more conformal. In the extremities, bone and subcutaneous doses were reduced by up to 20%. A conformal-IMRT comparative planning study has been reported for a large extraskeletal chondrosarcoma of the extremity.[61] Not surprisingly, IMRT produced excellent conformal treatment plans for this complex target volume, with less dose to the bone than the 3-D photon plan. Hong and colleagues[62] performed treatment-planning comparisons of IMRT and 3-D conformal RT for 10 patients with STS of the thigh. They were able to document a reduction in femur dose without compromise in tumor coverage. In addition, IMRT reduced dose inhomogeneity (ie, hot spots) in the surrounding soft tissues and skin.

In a single-institution retrospective study, Alektiar and colleagues[9] recently reported on a series of 41 adult patients with STS of the extremity treated with limb-sparing surgery and IMRT. In their cohort, 51% had positive or close (<1-mm) margins, and 68% had tumors greater than 10 cm. At a median follow-up of 35 months, an encouragingly low rate of complications was observed, with 4.8% developing fractures and 32% developing edema (the majority of whom had grade 1 edema). The 5-year actuarial LC rate was 94%. Both the toxicities and LC rates reported in this study are comparable to those achieved with 3-D conformal RT techniques.

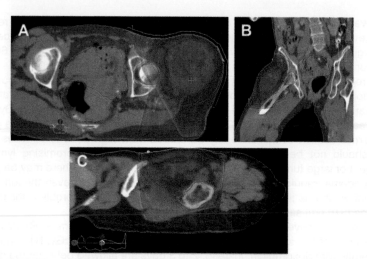

Fig. 4. Axial IMRT treatment plan—(*A*) axial, (*B*) coronal, and (*C*) sagittal—for a 71-year-old woman with a 12-cm right proximal thigh STS involving the subcutaneous tissue overlying the left hip as well as the lateral aspect of the rectus femoris and small portion of the vastus lateralis. IMRT was used to better spare the hip joint and the perineum. (*Courtesy of* Brian Napolitano, BS, CMD, Massachusetts General Hospital, Boston, MA.)

IMRT treatment plans, however, often have localized areas within the high-dose volumes, where dose inhomogeneities can be in the range of 10% to 15% above the prescription dose. Because there can also be dose inhomogeneities in the range of 5% below the target dose, treatment plans may be normalized to the 95% isodose line, meaning that selected areas of the treatment volume are receiving daily fractions and total doses of 15% to 20% above the target dose. Depending on the location of these hot spots, there can be unanticipated acute normal tissue toxicity.[63] Because of the multiple field angles used with IMRT, a greater volume of the extremity receives some RT dose, albeit in the low-dose to moderate-dose range. Although early experience suggests acceptable overall levels of late toxicity,[40] further study and longer follow-up are required to determine whether there are late effects specifically attributable to these focal areas of high dose or the larger volume of normal tissue exposed to these low to moderate doses. The group at Memorial Sloan-Kettering Cancer Center[40] recently adopted IMRT (over brachytherapy) as the preferred approach for adjuvant RT.

Proton Beam RT

The rationale for the use of protons (or other charged particles) rather than photons (ie, radiographs, which have traditionally been used for RT) is the approximately 60% reduction in radiation dose to normal tissue with protons. Protons and other charged particles deposit little energy in tissue until near the end of the proton range, where the residual energy is lost over a short distance, resulting in a steep rise in the absorbed dose, known as the Bragg peak (**Fig. 5**).[64,65] The Bragg peak is too narrow for practical clinical applications, so for the irradiation of most tumors, the beam energy is modulated by superimposing several Bragg peaks of descending energies (ranges) and weights to create a region of uniform dose over the depth of the target; these extended regions of uniform dose are called spread-out Bragg peaks (see **Fig. 5**). Although the beam modulation to spread out the Bragg peaks increases the entrance dose, the proton dose distribution is still characterized by a lower-dose region in normal tissue

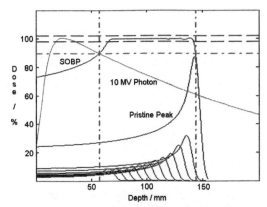

Fig. 5. Depth-dose distributions for a spread-out Bragg peak (SOBP) (red), its constituent pristine Bragg peaks (blue), and a 10-MV photon beam (black). The SOBP dose distribution is created by adding the contributions of individually modulated pristine Bragg peaks. The penetration depth, or range, measured as the depth of the distal 90% of plateau dose, of the SOBP dose distribution is determined by the range of the most distal pristine peak (labeled "Pristine Peak"). The dashed lines (black) indicate the clinically acceptable variation in the plateau dose of ±2%. The dot–dashed lines (green) indicate the 90% dose and spatial, range and modulation width intervals. The SOBP dose distribution of even a single field can provide complete target volume coverage in depth and lateral dimensions in sharp contrast to a single-field photon dose distribution; only a composite set of photon fields can deliver a clinical target dose distribution. The single photon field shown has a higher dose proximal to the tumor and deposits additional dose beyond the tumor. Note the absence of dose beyond the distal fall-off edge of the SOBP. (*Reprinted from* Levin WP, Kooy H, Loeffler JS, et al. Proton beam therapy. Br J Cancer 2005;93:849–54; with permission.)

proximal to the tumor, a uniform high-dose region in the tumor, and zero dose beyond the range of the deepest Bragg peak, which is usually just beyond the tumor target.

Although protons have been extensively used for sarcomas of the skull base and spine/paraspinal tissues, there may be opportunities to use protons with significant sparing of normal tissues in some patients with extremity STS (**Fig. 6**). Large, medial proximal thigh lesions can be effectively treated with sparing of the femur, hip joint, genitalia, and anorectal tissue. Lesions around the shoulder can be treated without irradiating the lung apex or shoulder joint. With the recent completion of proton beam facilities at major sarcoma centers in the United States (Massachusetts General Hospital, MD Anderson Cancer Center, University of Florida, and University of Pennsylvania) and Europe (Paul Scherrer Institute in Switzerland and Institut Curie in France as well as other centers in France, Italy, Sweden, and Germany), it is anticipated that a larger proportion of STS patients will be treated with protons.

Neoadjuvant Doxorubicin-Based Chemotherapy Plus RT

Eilber and colleagues, at the University of California, Los Angeles,[66] popularized preoperative regional chemotherapy and RT followed by limb salvage surgery in patients with high-grade STSs. They were able to achieve a high rate of primary limb salvage, low rate of LR (approximately 9%), and long-term survival in 65% of patients. The current regimen consists of doxorubicin (30 mg per day for 3 days) followed by RT given at 28 Gy in 8 fractions. Several other groups using this regimen have also obtained low rates of LR with varying degrees of toxicity.[67] It is not clear if intra-arterial administration provides added benefit over intravenous doxorubicin.

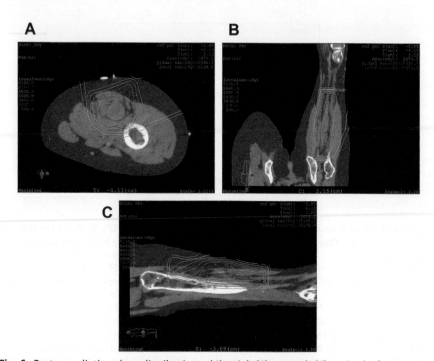

Fig. 6. Proton radiation dose distribution—(*A*) axial, (*B*) coronal, (*C*) sagittal—for a patient with a radiation-associated malignant peripheral nerve sheath tumor arising in the setting of prior RT 18 years earlier for Ewing sarcoma of the femur, metastatic at diagnosis. As it was expected to be difficult to achieve wide margins, preoperative radiation was recommended. Preoperative protons were used to reduce the radiation dose to the normal tissues in the thigh. (*Courtesy of* Judy Adams, CMD, Massachusetts General Hospital, Boston, MA.)

One study comparing these 2 methods of administration found that the intra-arterial route was thought associated with a higher incidence of complications but no improvement in survival or function.[68] Another report evaluated 2 separate protocols using preoperative treatment with intravenous doxorubicin and ifosfamide with or without intra-arterial cisplatin; the histologic response and LR rates after surgery were better with the all-intravenous regimen.[69]

Combination intravenous chemotherapy regimens, such as mesna, doxorubicin, ifosfamide, and dacarbazine (MAID), may provide better antitumor activity than single-agent doxorubicin. Interesting results have been noted with neoadjuvant MAID plus RT.[20,70] The experience with preoperative MAID chemotherapy interdigitated with 44 Gy RT and followed by surgery, postoperative MAID, and further RT (16 Gy) for those with positive margins was reported in a series of 48 patients with high-grade extremity STS greater than or equal to 8 cm.[20] Despite the low objective response rate to preoperative therapy (partial response in 5 and stable disease in 36), all patients were able to undergo limb-sparing surgery initially, with 7 having positive margins. Median tumor necrosis was 95%, suggesting that conventional imaging in this setting may underestimate the degree of response to therapy. Hospitalization for febrile neutropenia occurred in 25% of patients at some time during treatment. Wound healing complications developed in 14 of 48 MAID patients (29%). One MAID patient developed late fatal myelodysplasia. The 5-year rates of LC (92% vs 86%), freedom from distant metastases (75% vs 44%), disease-free survival (70% vs 42%), and OS (87% vs 58%) all compared favorably with the outcomes of a cohort of historical control patients who were matched for tumor size, grade, patient age, and era of treatment.

There were similar results when this regimen was used in a multicenter United States cooperative group trial, in which 66 patients (64 of whom were analyzed) with primary high-grade STS 8 cm or larger in diameter received a modified MAID regimen plus granulocyte colony-stimulating factor and RT, followed by resection and postoperative chemotherapy.[70] Although preoperative chemotherapy and RT was successfully completed by 79% and 89% of patients, respectively, grade 4 hematological and nonhematological toxicity was experienced by 78% and 19% of patients, respectively. Grade 3 or grade 4 skin toxicity was noted in 34%. The limb preservation rate was 92%. With a median follow-up of 2.75 years, the estimated 3-year OS, disease-free survival, and locoregional control rates were 75%, 56%, and 82%, respectively. Three patients (5%) experienced fatal grade 5 toxicities, among whom 2 developed late myelodysplasia and 1 developed infection. It remains to be confirmed in randomized studies whether these aggressive interdigitated approaches offer benefit to the subgroup of patients with large, high-grade sarcomas, who are at the highest risk of treatment failure.

Combining Adjuvant RT with Adjuvant Chemotherapy

Adjuvant chemotherapy is standard treatment of rhabdomyosarcoma,[71,72] osteosarcoma, and Ewing sarcoma[73] but is not definitively established in other adult STSs.[74,75] This topic is discussed in the article by Ravi and Patel elsewhere in this issue. The patients most commonly receiving adjuvant chemotherapy, those with deep, intermediate or high-grade STS greater than 5 cm, are generally patients who are likely to also require adjuvant RT. For these patients, chemotherapy has been sequenced with RT in a variety of schedules without any current standard approach. For nearly all of these, concurrent administration of standard doses and schedules of adriamycin, gemcitabine, actinomycin D, and other potent radiosensitizers with standard RT fraction schedules has generally not been done to avoid excessive acute and potentially late normal tissue toxicity. Some of these agents, however, have been combined with RT using altered schedules or doses (discussed previously), such as that popularized by Eilber and colleagues,[66] the interdigitated MAID chemoradiation studies,[20,70] and those in other experimental studies using altered chemotherapy and/or RT dose delivery schemes.[76]

Soft Tissue Sarcomas of the Hand and Foot

The 5-year survival rate for STS of the hand and foot is approximately 80%, better than that for other extremity sites.[77–80] This is likely related to the smaller size of these lesions at presentation. With surgical excision and the use of adjunctive RT when the minimum surgical margin is narrow (<2 mm), limb amputation can be avoided as primary therapy in most patients and up to two-thirds of patients can retain a normal or fairly normal extremity.

Wound Healing After Surgery and RT

In general, the use of adjunctive RT is associated with a higher frequency of wound complications. Precise quantification of the impact of RT on wound healing is difficult, however, because of the significant complications seen with surgery alone. In addition, there is much heterogeneity among patients with STS with respect to anatomic site, histologic type, lesion size, prior surgery, medical comorbidities, and age. The use of adjunctive RT can also be associated with joint stiffness, edema, and decreased range of motion.[6,81] In one trial, extremity RT resulted in significantly worse limb strength, edema, and range of motion than with surgery alone for extremity STS, but the symptoms were transient and did not affect global quality of life.[6]

Preoperative RT and Wound Complications

Preoperative RT is associated with a higher incidence of acute wound complications.[7] In the randomized study of preoperative versus postoperative RT, a significantly higher percentage of preoperatively treated patients had acute wound complications (35% vs 17%). In another series of 202 patients undergoing preoperative RT, the overall wound complication rate was 37%.[81] One patient died with necrotizing fasciitis and 33 (17%) required secondary surgery, including 6 (3%) who required amputation. In a recent retrospective study of 173 patients, major wound complications were more likely to occur in the lower extremity than in the upper extremity.[82] In this cohort, 59% of whom also received preoperative chemotherapy, the rate of major wound complications was 32% after preoperative RT. In another report, wound morbidity was 25% (4 of 16) in patients treated with preoperative external beam RT plus BRT at the time of surgery but only 5% (2 of 40) in those treated postoperatively with BRT followed by external beam RT.[37]

Brachytherapy and Wound Complications

The use of perioperative BRT may increase the incidence of wound complications. In one study of 105 patients with extremity and truncal sarcomas, major wound complications occurred in 9 of 41 (22%) patients treated with BRT compared with 2 of 64 (3%) non–BRT-treated patients.[83] Patients treated with BRT also had a higher total number of complications as well as a higher combined frequency of major and moderate wound complications (44% vs 14%), and a longer time to wound healing (189 days vs 49 days).

The findings were different in a randomized trial of adjuvant BRT versus no BRT, however, in 164 patients with resected extremity or truncal STS.[83] The incidence of serious wound complications was not significantly increased in the group receiving BRT (24% vs 14%, $P = .133$), but the incidence of wound reoperation was increased (6% vs 0%).[38]

Strategies to Reduce Wound Morbidity

Based on the available literature, the following strategies are suggested to reduce acute wound morbidity in patients being treated with preoperative RT[81] or perioperative BRT[38]:

- Gentle handling of tissue during surgery
- Meticulous attention to achieving hemostasis before wound closure
- Avoidance of closure under tension
- Elimination of all wound dead space, using a rotated flap to fill the space, if necessary
- Wound drainage with tubes remaining in place until drainage has decreased to satisfactory levels
- Use of compression dressings
- Immobilization of the affected part for approximately 7 days
- Delineation of a subgroup of patients in whom postoperative boost dose can be omitted, which includes patients with negative margins and no tumor cut-through, complete tumor necrosis, or absence of tumor in the resection

specimen and perhaps some patients with low-grade tumors and planned, focally positive margins.[52]

Functional Outcome

There are increasing data available on the functional outcome of patients undergoing limb salvage procedures.[27,59,84,85] The majority of patients have good or excellent functional outcome. In one series of 88 patients treated with surgery and either preoperative or postoperative RT, 68 had acceptable functional results, and 61 returned to work.[27] Large tumors, neural sacrifice, proximal thigh tumors, and postoperative complications were associated with poor outcome. Subcutaneous tumors have a more favorable functional outcome.[86] In a single institution series of 145 patients who underwent limb-sparing surgery plus RT, long-term treatment complications included bone fracture in 6%, contracture in 20%, significant edema in 19%, moderate to severe decrease in muscle strength in 20%, requirement for a cane or crutch in 7%, and tissue induration in 57%.[59] Of these patients, 3 (2%) required amputations for treatment-related complications. The percentage of patients ambulating without assistive devices and with mild or no pain was 84%. Higher doses of RT, a long RT portal, and irradiation of more than 75% of the extremity diameter were associated with increased morbidity. Another study examined issues related to quality of life in patients with STS of the lower limb.[85] Although RT was associated with reduced muscle power and range of motion compared with surgery alone, most patients retained good to excellent limb function and quality of life.

The functional outcome is often not as good in patients requiring amputation. In a matched case-control study of patients with lower extremity STS undergoing amputation (n = 12) or a limb-sparing approach (n = 24), there was a trend toward increased disability and handicap for those in the amputation group.[84] Of the 12 amputees, 7 reported ongoing problems with the soft tissue overlying the stump. A Swedish study showed similar results with amputees having a significantly lower Musculoskeletal Tumor Society (MSTS) scoring system score than those with limb-sparing surgery (P<.001), but there was no difference for the Toronto Extremity Salvage Score (TESS). Tumor localization above knee level resulted in significantly lower MSTS scores and TESS (P = .003 and P = .02, respectively). There were no significant differences in quality of life between amputees and those with limb-sparing surgery except in physical functioning; 11% of all patients did not work or study. In multivariate analysis, amputation, tumor location above the knee and having muscular pain were associated with low physical function.[87] In the few studies that have assessed quality-of-life issues in STS patients treated with amputation and chemotherapy compared with patients who underwent limb salvage with RT and chemotherapy, contrary to expectations, there were no significant differences in measures of psychological outcome.[88,89] Thus, a psychological advantage of limb-salvage surgery over amputation has yet to be demonstrated.

Treatment of Local Recurrence

Approximately 10% to 15% of patients with extremity STS who are treated with complete resection and adjuvant RT develop a local tumor failure, the majority within the first 2 years.[26,27,51,90] The approach to patients with an isolated LR is similar to that for those with primary disease, with some modifications. As with primary treatment, the goal is to achieve tumor control, and, if possible, limb salvage with conservative resection. Approximately 10% to 25% of patients with LR disease, however, require amputation.[91–93] Surgery is an important component of successful salvage therapy.[91] For patients whose primary treatment was surgery alone, re-excision combined with adjuvant RT is the treatment of choice. If RT was used as part of the primary treatment, further RT may not be possible because the maximal tolerance for adjacent normal tissues would have to be exceeded, resulting in a significant risk for problems with wound healing or radiation fibrosis. Additional RT given by BRT (mean dose 47.2 Gy) has been used, however, in some of these patients, with 52% LC and a 33% disease-free survival rates in one series of 26 patients.[94]

Optimal treatment of LR may require both surgery and RT. This was illustrated in one report of salvage therapy using surgery alone or surgery plus reirradiation for 25 patients with LR extremity STS.[91] In the 18 patients undergoing surgery alone, 11 were treated by a conservative procedure and 7 required amputation. Of these 18 patients, 7 relapsed. Of the 10 patients treated with surgery plus RT, none experienced relapse with a median follow-up of 24 months. Six patients (60%) experienced significant wound healing complications, but 3 recovered completely.

Treatment of Locally Advanced Soft Tissue Sarcoma

In patients with advanced STS in whom the tumor has progressed to a point that the functional morbidity of an attempted limb salvage resection is too great for the patient, nonamputative treatment options depend on the site of tumor involvement. For patients with this type of disease limited to the extremity, isolated limb perfusion protocols have been applied with some success. Selected patients can also have their tumors controlled with RT with or without chemotherapy, especially when the tumors are small. For patients treated with a dose of 6400 cGy or greater, Tepper and Suit[32] reported control of unresected STSs in 87.5% of cases of tumors that less than 5 cm in diameter. Treatment was less effective for larger tumors, with LC falling to 53% for lesions 5 cm to 10 cm diameter (53%) and 30% for those greater than 10 cm. Kepka and colleagues[1] recently updated and expanded this experience, reporting on the efficacy of RT on 112 patients with unresected STS. For patients receiving 63 Gy or more, LC at 5 years was 72.4% in patients with lesions 5 cm or less, 42.4% for lesions 5 cm to 10 cm, and 25.4% for lesions greater than 10 cm.

Several centers have reported LC rates of approximately 50% with fast neutron irradiation of inoperable STSs.[95–97] In addition, several RT sensitizers have been used to treat patients with extensive STS with promising early preliminary results.[98–100] Trabectedin (ET-743), a novel antitumor agent, has also shown promise in advanced STS, both as a single agent and in combination with other agents.[101,102]

Summary: Extremity and Truncal Soft Tissue Sarcomas

Treatment of extremity STS requires individual tailoring of the approach because of the wide variety of clinical situations that can arise from tumors that involve various anatomic sites with a range of histologies of differing grades and sizes. Nevertheless, the following suggestions can serve as useful guides. Surgery is always indicated, but the use of adjuvant therapy can vary according to the anatomic site, size, and histologic grade.

- In general, patients with superficial, low-grade tumors that are less than 5 cm in diameter can be treated with surgical excision alone when negative margins of greater than 1 cm or an investing fascial barrier or other high-quality tissue plane, such as periosteum, is resected with the tumor. Such patients can expect excellent LC and survival rates approximating 90%.
- In patients with intermediate-grade lesions, surgical excision with negative margins in combination with RT has achieved excellent LC with OS rates approximating 80%.

- For larger, deep-seated tumors, preoperative RT or postoperative RT seem to have similar efficacy in preventing LR, although postoperative RT generally treats a larger target volume and requires higher doses to the tumor bed. Acute wound healing complications are higher with preoperative RT for lower extremity lesions, but generally irreversible late complications, including grades 3 and 4 fibrosis, are more common in those patients receiving postoperative RT.
- In patients with high-grade STS greater than 5 cm, excellent LC can be achieved with surgery and RT, but at least 50% of these patients develop metastatic disease. In this setting, the use of neoadjuvant chemotherapy may benefit some and should be considered in the context of a clinical trial, to be followed by definitive surgery combined with either preoperative or postoperative RT or BRT.
- BRT can provide excellent LC and functional results in appropriately selected patients.

RETROPERITONEAL SARCOMAS

Approximately 10% to 15% of STSs arise in the retroperitoneum.[103,104] These tumors are often asymptomatic and identified on imaging studies for unrelated complaints. In other cases, patients may present with a palpable abdominal mass or with symptoms, such as abdominal pain or lower extremity neurologic symptoms.[104,105] Approximately 10% to 20% of patients are found to have distant metastases on initial presentation.[106]

Because the retroperitoneum can often accommodate large tumors without symptoms, the average size of tumors in large series is often greater than 10 cm.[105,106] Approximately two-thirds of tumors are either liposarcomas or leiomyosarcomas, with the remaining tumors distributed among a large variety of histologic subtypes.[105] Retroperitoneal liposarcomas are further classified into well-differentiated, dedifferentiated, and myxoid/round cell subtypes. In the largest series of retroperitoneal liposarcomas (n = 177), 56% were well differentiated, 37% dedifferentiated, and 7% myxoid/round cell.[107] Approximately 40% of tumors are low-grade and the remaining 60% are intermediate-grade or high-grade.[103] Low-grade tumors uncommonly metastasize, whereas intermediate-grade and high-grade tumors can metastasize to the lung and liver.

Most unifocal tumors in the retroperitoneum that do not arise from adjacent organs are either benign soft tissue tumors (eg, schwannomas) or sarcomas. Other malignancies in the differential diagnosis include primary germ cell tumor, metastatic testicular cancer, and lymphoma. After a careful history and physical examination, radiologic assessment of these tumors is usually performed with an abdomen and pelvic CT scan. Liposarcomas often have a characteristic appearance, with large areas of abnormal fat (well-differentiated liposarcoma) often containing higher-density nodules (dedifferentiated liposarcoma). Leiomyosarcomas appear as heterogeneous solid tumors. MRI scans may be helpful in delineating tumors from adjacent soft tissues, nerves, or major blood vessels but are usually not necessary. To evaluate for metastatic disease, the abdomen CT is adequate in evaluating the liver. Patients with intermediate-grade and high-grade tumors should have a chest CT to evaluate for lung metastases. A chest radiograph is obtained for low-grade tumors.

The primary treatment of the LC of these tumors is surgical resection. The optimal goal of surgical resection is complete gross resection with microscopically negative margins. Even complete gross resection can be difficult to obtain, however; complete resection rates in large series range from 54% to 67%.[105,106,108] In approximately three-quarters of cases, complete gross resection requires resection of adjacent viscera.[105] For tumors abutting the kidney, the renal capsule can often be resected in lieu of a formal nephrectomy given that 75% of kidneys resected in one series showed no renal capsule, parenchyma, or vessel invasion.[109]

The ability to obtain negative microscopic margins for large retroperitoneal STS is also difficult. These tumors are surrounded by a pseudocapsule that is often infiltrated by microscopic disease, and dissection with a normal tissue margin away from the pseudocapsule is difficult, especially along the posterior aspect of the tumor where it abuts the retroperitoneal fat and musculature. A positive or negative microscopic margin was not a prognostic factor for LR in the largest series of retroperitoneal STS from Memorial Sloan-Kettering Cancer Center.[105] Many large retroperitoneal STSs, however, considered to have negative microscopic margins most likely have positive margins in areas not specifically examined pathologically. Prognostic factors for LR in that series were incomplete gross resection, high grade, and liposarcoma histology.

Controversy exists as to the optimal role of RT for LC of retroperitoneal STS. Although there are some data to suggest a benefit for postoperative RT,[106] those who advocate RT usually prefer that RT be delivered preoperatively.[104] With the tumor still in place, the margin around the tumor at risk of LR is more clearly defined, and the effective RT dose to control microscopic disease is likely lower. The American College of Surgeons Oncology Group opened a phase III randomized trial of preoperative RT and surgery versus surgery alone for retroperitoneal STS in 2004. Unfortunately, this study was closed because of poor accrual and thus did not provide any level 1 evidence on the efficacy of neoadjuvant RT.

Petersen and colleagues[110] reviewed their experience at the Mayo Clinic with 43 patients who received external beam RT (usually preoperatively) and intraoperative RT. LC was 75% at 5 years. Approximately one-fifth of patients had IORT toxicity, including gastrointestinal fistula, neuropathy, and ureteral injury. The University of Toronto Sarcoma Group treated 55 patients with retroperitoneal STS with either preoperative external beam RT or BRT and found that external beam RT (median dose 45 Gy) was well tolerated whereas BRT to the upper abdomen was associated with significant toxicity.[111]

In a report from the author's institution, 29 patients were treated with preoperative RT to a median dose of 45 Gy and then underwent complete gross resection.[112] Intraoperative RT 10 Gy to 20 Gy was delivered to 16 patients and no IORT was delivered to 13 patients. LC at 5 years was 83% for patients who received both preoperative RT and IORT and 61% for those who received only preoperative RT. Significant toxicity from IORT occurred in 4 patients, including neuropathy, ureteral stricture, and vaginal fistula. More recently, the author and colleagues have incorporated the use of preoperative IMRT and/or proton beam RT along with resection and IORT for retroperitoneal STS and have found that these techniques allow for dose escalation to areas at risk while decreasing the dose to adjacent organs.[11]

In the extremity, the LC of STSs treated with RT and total gross resection with positive microscopic margin is approximately 75%.[27,51,113,114] Typically, positive microscopic margins are treated with a boost of postoperative RT to a total dose of approximately 66 Gy to 68 Gy. It seems reasonable to assume that total gross resection of retroperitoneal STSs along with adequate doses of RT could achieve LC rates similar to that seen for extremity STSs resected with positive microscopic margins. The availability of intensity modulated RT techniques, proton beam RT, and IORT may facilitate the efficacy and minimize morbidity of adjuvant RT for the retroperitoneal tumors and translate into improved LC.

The addition of chemotherapy to current RT strategies may potentially improve the LC of retroperitoneal STS and may have some impact on distant disease. A few small series have been reported. In one study, 16 patients were treated with iododeoxyuridine and RT with only 3 patients experiencing grade 4 toxicity (vomiting).[115] Eleven patients went on to resection and 4 patients had an LR. Pisters and colleagues[76] at the MD Anderson Cancer Center treated 35 patients in a phase I trial of doxorubicin and escalating doses of external beam RT. Two of 11 patients had grade 3 or 4 toxicity at the highest dose of external beam RT (50.4 Gy). IORT was delivered to 22 of 29 patients who subsequently underwent surgery. LC results have not yet been published.

REFERENCES

1. Kepka L, DeLaney TF, Goldberg SI, et al. Results of radiation therapy for unresected soft tissue sarcomas. Int J Radiat Oncol Biol Phys 2005;63:852.
2. Baldini EH, Goldberg J, Jenner C, et al. Long-term outcomes after functon-sparing surgery without radiotherapy for soft tissue sarcoma of the extemities and trunk. J Clin Oncol 1999;17:3252.
3. White LM, Wunder JS, Bell RS, et al. Histologic assessment of peritumoral edema in soft tissue sarcoma. Int J Radiat Oncol Biol Phys 2005;61:1439.
4. Markhede G, Angervall L, Stener B. A multivariate analysis of the prognosis after surgical treatment of malignant soft-tissue tumors. Cancer 1982;49:1721.
5. Pisters PW, Harrison LB, Leung DH, et al. Long-term results of a prospective randomized trial of adjuvant brachytherapy in soft tissue sarcoma. J Clin Oncol 1996;14:859.
6. Yang JC, Chang AE, Baker AR, et al. Randomized prospective study of the benefit of adjuvant radiation therapy in the treatment of soft tissue sarcomas of the extremity. J Clin Oncol 1998;16:197.
7. O'Sullivan B, Davis AM, Turcotte R, et al. Preoperative versus postoperative radiotherapy in soft-tissue sarcoma of the limbs: a randomized trial. Lancet 2002;359:2235.
8. Davis AM, O'Sullivan B, Turcotte R, et al. Late radiation morbidity following randomization to preoperative versus postoperative radiotherapy in extremity soft tissue sarcoma. Radiother Oncol 2005;75:48.
9. Alektiar KM, Brennan MF, Healey JH, et al. Impact of intensity-modulated radiation therapy on local control in primary soft-tissue sarcoma of the extremity. J Clin Oncol 2008;26:3440.
10. Griffin AM, Euler CI, Sharpe MB, et al. Radiation planning comparison for superficial tissue avoidance in radiotherapy for soft tissue sarcoma of the lower extremity. Int J Radiat Oncol Biol Phys 2007;67:847.
11. Yoon SS, Chen YL, Kirsch DG, et al. Proton-beam, intensity-modulated, and/or intraoperative electron radiation therapy combined with aggressive anterior surgical resection for retroperitoneal sarcomas. Ann Surg Oncol 2010;17:1515.
12. Gustafson P, Dreinhofer KE, Rydholm A. Soft tissue sarcoma should be treated at a tumor center. A comparison of quality of surgery in 375 patients. Acta Orthop Scand 1994;65:47.
13. Simon MA, Enneking WF. The management of soft-tissue sarcomas of the extremities. J Bone Joint Surg Am 1976;58:317.
14. Rosenberg SA, Tepper J, Glatstein E, et al. The treatment of soft-tissue sarcomas of the extremities: prospective randomized evaluations of (1) limb-sparing surgery plus radiation therapy compared with amputation and (2) the role of adjuvant chemotherapy. Ann Surg 1982;196:305.
15. Rydholm A, Berg NO, Gullber B, et al. Epidemiology of soft tissue sarcoma in the locomotor system. Acta Pathol Microbiol Immunol Scand A 1984;92:363.

16. Lindberg RD, Martin RG, Romsdahl MM, et al. Conservative surgery and postoperative radiotherapy in 300 adults with soft-tissue sarcomas. Cancer 1981;47:2391.
17. Suit HD, Russell WO, Martin RG. Sarcoma of soft tissue: clinical and histopathologic parameters and response to treatment. Cancer 1975;35:1478.
18. Abbatucci JS, Boulier N, de Ranieri J, et al. Local control and survival in soft tissue sarcomas of the limbs, trunk walls and head and neck: a study of 113 cases. Int J Radiat Oncol Biol Phys 1986;12:579.
19. Brant TA, Parsons JT, Marcus RB, et al. Preoperative irradiation for soft tissue sarcomas of the trunk and extremities in adults. Int J Radiat Oncol Biol Phys 1990;19.
20. DeLaney TF, Spiro IJ, Suit HD, et al. Neoadjuvant chemotherapy and radiotherapy for large extremity soft-tissue sarcomas. Int J Radiat Oncol Biol Phys 2003;56:1117.
21. Eilber FR, Eckardt J. Surgical management of soft tissue sarcomas. Semin Oncol 1997;24:526.
22. Harrison LB, Franzese F, Gaynor JJ, et al. Long-term results of a prospective randomized trial of adjuvant brachytherapy in the management of completely resected soft tissue sarcomas of the extremity and superficial trunk. Int J Radiat Oncol Biol Phys 1993;27:259.
23. Karakousis CP, Emrich LJ, Rao U, et al. Feasibility of limb salvage and survival in soft tissue sarcomas. Cancer 1986;57:484.
24. Potter DA, Glenn J, Kinsella T, et al. Patterns of recurrence in patients with high-grade soft tissue sarcomas. J Clin Oncol 1985;3:353.
25. Wilson AN, Davis A, Bell RS, et al. Local control of soft tissue sarcoma of the extremity: the experience of a multidisciplinary sarcoma group with definitive surgery and radiotherapy. Eur J Cancer 1994;30A:746.
26. Karakousis CP, Driscoll DL. Treatment and local control of primary extremity soft tissue sarcomas. J Surg Oncol 1999;71:155.
27. LeVay J, O'Sullivan B, Catton C, et al. Outcome and prognostic factors in soft tissue sarcoma in the adult. Int J Radiat Oncol Biol Phys 1993;27:1091.
28. Williard WC, Hajdu SI, Casper ES, et al. Comparison of amputation with limb-sparing operations for adult soft tissue sarcoma of the extremity. Ann Surg 1992;215:389.
29. Rydholm A, Gustafson P, Rooser B, et al. Limb-sparing surgery without radiotherapy based on anatomic location of soft tissue sarcoma. J Clin Oncol 1991;9:1757.
30. Pisters PW, Pollock RE, Lewis VO, et al. Long-term results of prospective trial of surgery alone with selective use of radiation for patients with T1 extremity and trunk soft tissue sarcomas. Ann Surg 2007;246:675.
31. Ruka W, Taghian A, Gioioso D, et al. Comparison between the in vitro intrinsic radiation sensitivity of human soft tissue sarcoma and breast cancer cell lines. J Surg Oncol 1996;61:290.
32. Tepper JE, Suit HD. Radiation therapy alone for sarcoma of soft tissue. Cancer 1985;56:475.
33. Todoroki T, Suit HD. Therapeutic advantage in preoperative single-dose radiation combined with conservative and radical surgery in different-size murine fibrosarcomas. J Surg Oncol 1985;29:207.
34. O'Sullivan B, Davis A, Bell R, et al. Phase III randomized trial of pre-operative versus post-operative radiotherapy in the curative management of extremity soft tissue sarcoma. A Canadian Sarcoma Group and NCI Canada Clinical Trials Group study. Proc Am Soc Clin Oncol 1999;18:2066a.

35. Davis AM, O'Sullivan B, Bell RS, et al. Function and health status outcomes in a randomized trial comparing preoperative and postoperative radiotherapy in extremity soft tissue sarcoma. J Clin Oncol 2002;20:4472.
36. O'Sullivan B, Davis AM, Turcotte R, et al. Five-year results of a randomized phase III trial of pre-operative vs. post-operative radiotherapy in extremity soft tissue sarcoma. Proc Am Soc Clin Oncol 2004;23:815.
37. Schray MF, Gunderson LL, Sim FH, et al. Soft tissue sarcomas. Integration of brachytherapy, resection, and external irradiation. Cancer 1990;66:451.
38. Alektiar KM, Zelefsky MJ, Brennan MF. Morbidity of adjuvant brachytherapy in soft tissue sarcoma of the extremity and superficial trunk. Int J Radiat Oncol Biol Phys 2000;47:1273.
39. Panagopoulos I, Hoglund M, Mertens F, et al. Fusion of EWS and CHOP genes in myxoid liposarcoma. Oncogene 1996;12:489.
40. Alektiar KM, Brennan MF, Singer S. Local control comparison of adjuvant brachytherapy to intensity-modulated radiotherapy in primary high-grade sarcoma of the extremity. Cancer 2011;117:3229.
41. Kretzler A, Molls M, Gradinger R, et al. Intraoperative radiotherapy of soft tissue sarcoma of the extremity. Perioperative fractionated high-dose rate brachytherapy in the treatment of soft tissue sarcomas. Strahlenther Onkol 2004;180:365.
42. Nag S, Shasha D, Janjan N, et al. The American Brachytherapy Society recommendations for brachytherapy of soft tissue sarcomas. Int J Radiat Oncol Biol Phys 2001;49:1033.
43. Petera J, Neumanova R, Odrazka K, et al. Perioperative fractionated high-dose rate brachytherapy in the treatment of soft tissue sarcomas. Neoplasma 2004;51:59.
44. Beltrami G, Rudiger HA, Mela MM, et al. Limb salvage surgery in combination with brachytherapy and external beam radiation for high-grade soft tissue sarcomas. Eur J Surg Oncol 2008;34:811.
45. Tepper J, Rosenberg SA, Glatstein E. Radiation therapy technique in soft tissue sarcomas of the extremity–policies of treatment at the National Cancer Institute. Int J Radiat Oncol Biol Phys 1982;8:263.
46. Suit HD, Mankin HJ, Wood WC, et al. Treatment of the patient with stage M0 sarcoma of soft tissue. J Clin Oncol 1988;6:854.
47. Mundt AJ, Awan A, Sibley GS, et al. Conservative surgery and adjuvant radiation therapy in the management of adult soft tissue sarcoma of the extremities: clinical and radiobiological results. Int J Radiat Oncol Biol Phys 1995; 32:977.
48. Cleator SJ, Cottril C, Harmer C. Pattern of local recurrence after conservative surgery and radiotherapy for soft tissue sarcoma. Sarcoma 2001;5:83.
49. Kim B, Chen YL, Kirsch DG, et al. An effective preoperative three-dimensional radiotherapy target volume for extremity soft tissue sarcoma and the effect of margin width on local control. Int J Radiat Oncol Biol Phys 2010;77:843.
50. Haglund KE, Raut CP, Nascimento AF, et al. Recurrence patterns and survival for ptients with Intermediate- and high-grade myxofibrosarcoma. Int J Radiat Oncol Biol Phys 2012;82:361.
51. Sadoski C, Suit HD, Rosenberg A, et al. Preoperative radiation, surgical margins, and local control of extremity sarcomas of soft tissues. J Surg Oncol 1993;52:223.
52. Al Yami A, Griffin AM, Ferguson PC, et al. Positive surgical margins in soft tissue sarcoma treated with preoperative radiation: is a postoperative boost necessary? Int J Radiat Oncol Biol Phys 2010;77:1191.

53. Zagars GK, Ballo MT. Significance of dose in postoperative radiotherapy for soft tissue sarcoma. Int J Radiat Oncol Biol Phys 2003;56:473.
54. Fein DA, Lee WR, Lanciano RM, et al. Management of extremity soft tissue sarcomas with limb-sparing surgery and postoperative irradiation: do total dose, overall treatment time, and the surgery-radiotherapy interval impact on local control? Int J Radiat Oncol Biol Phys 1995;32:969.
55. Bell RS, O'Sullivan B, Liu FF, et al. The surgical margin in soft tissue sarcoma. J Bone Joint Surg Am 1989;71:370.
56. Pao WJ, Pilepich MV. Postoperative radiotherapy in the treatment of extremity soft tissue sarcomas. Int J Radiat Oncol Biol Phys 1990;19:907.
57. Robinson M, Barr L, Fisher C, et al. Treatment of extremity soft tissue sarcomas with surgery and radiotherapy. Radiother Oncol 1990;18:221.
58. Robinson MH, Ball AB, Schofield J, et al. Preoperative radiotherapy for initially inoperable extremity soft tissue sarcomas. Clin Oncol (R Coll Radiol) 1992;4:36.
59. Stinson SF, DeLaney TF, Greenberg J, et al. Acute and long term effects on limb function of combined modality limb sparing therapy for extremity soft tissue sarcomas. Int J Radiat Oncol Biol Phys 1991;21:1493.
60. Verhey LJ. Comparison of three-dimensional conformal radiation therapy and intensity-modulated radiation therapy systems. Semin Radiat Oncol 1999;9:78.
61. Chan MF, Chui CS, Schupak K, et al. The treatment of large extraskeletal chondrosarcoma of the leg: comparison of IMRT and conformal radiotherapy techniques. J Appl Clin Med Phys 2001;2:3.
62. Hong L, Alektiar KM, Hunt M, et al. Intensity-modulated radiotherapy for soft tissue sarcoma of the thigh. Int J Radiat Oncol Biol Phys 2004;59:752.
63. Lee N, Chuang C, Quivey JM, et al. Skin toxicity due to intensity-modulated radiotherapy for head-and-neck carcinoma. Int J Radiat Oncol Biol Phys 2002;53:630.
64. Austin-Seymour M, Munzenrider J, Goitein M, et al. Fractionated proton radiation therapy of chordoma and low grade chondrosarcoma of the base of skull. J Neurosurg 1989;70:13.
65. Wilson RR. Radiological uses of fast protons. Radiology 1946;47:487.
66. Eilber FC, Rosen G, Eckardt J, et al. Treatment-induced pathologic necrosis: a predictor of local recurrence and survival in patients receiving neoadjuvant therapy for high-grade extremity soft tissue sarcomas. J Clin Oncol 2001;19:3203.
67. Wanebo HJ, Temple WJ, Popp MB, et al. Preoperative regional therapy for extremity sarcoma. A tricenter update. Cancer 1995;75:2299.
68. Eilber F, Eckardt J, Rosen G, et al. Preoperative therapy for soft tissue sarcoma. Hematol Oncol Clin North Am 1995;9:817.
69. Merimsky O, Meller I, Issakov J, et al. Adriamycin-ifosfamide induction chemotherapy for extremity soft tissue sarcoma: comparison of two non-randomized protocols. Oncol Rep 1999;6:913.
70. Kraybill WG, Harris J, Spiro IJ, et al. Phase II study of neoadjuvant chemotherapy and radiation therapy in the management of high-risk, high-grade, soft tissue sarcomas of the extremities and body wall: radiation Therapy Oncology Group Trial 9514. J Clin Oncol 2006;24:619.
71. Bramwell V. The role of chemotherapy in the management of non-metastatic operable extremity osteosarcoma. Semin Oncol 1997;24:561.
72. Crist WM, Anderson JR, Meza JL, et al. Intergroup rhabdomyosarcoma study-IV: results for patients with nonmetastatic disease. J Clin Oncol 2001;19:3091.

73. Rosen G, Caparros B, Nirenberg A, et al. Ewing's sarcoma: ten-year experience with adjuvant chemotherapy. Cancer 1981;47:2204.
74. Antman KH. Adjuvant therapy of sarcomas of soft tissue. Semin Oncol 1997;24:556.
75. Scurr M, Judson I. Neoadjuvant and adjuvant therapy for extremity soft tissue sarcomas. Hematol Oncol Clin North Am 2005;19:489.
76. Pisters PW, Ballo MT, Fenstermacher MJ, et al. Phase I trial of preoperative concurrent doxorubicin and radiation therapy, surgical resection, and intraoperative electron-beam radiation therapy for patients with localized retroperitoneal sarcoma. J Clin Oncol 2003;21:3092.
77. Johnstone PA, Wexler LH, Venzon DJ, et al. Sarcomas of the hand and foot: analysis of local control and functional result with combined modality therapy in extremity preservation. Int J Radiat Oncol Biol Phys 1994;29:735.
78. Karakousis CP, De Young C, Driscoll DL. Soft tissue sarcomas of the hand and foot: management and survival. Ann Surg Oncol 1998;5:238.
79. Pradhan A, Cheung YC, Grimer RJ, et al. Soft-tissue sarcomas of the hand: oncological outcome and prognostic factors. J Bone Joint Surg Br 2008;90:209.
80. Talbert ML, Zagars GK, Sherman NE, et al. Conservative surgery and radiation therapy for soft tissue sarcoma of the wrist, hand, ankle, and foot. Cancer 1990; 66:2482.
81. Bujko K, Suit HD, Springfield DS, et al. Wound healing after surgery and preoperative radiation for sarcoma of soft tissues. Surg Gynecol Obstet 1992;176:124.
82. Tseng JF, Ballo MT, Langstein HN, et al. The effect of preoperative radiotherapy and reconstructive surgery on wound complications after resection of extremity soft-tissue sarcomas. Ann Surg Oncol 2006;13:1209.
83. Arbeit JM, Hilaris B, Brennan MF. Wound complications in the multimodality treatment of extremity and superficial truncal sarcomas. J Clin Oncol 1987; 5:480.
84. Davis AM, Devlin M, Griffin AM, et al. Functional outcome in amputation versus limb sparing of patients with lower extremity sarcoma: a matched case-control study. Arch Phys Med Rehabil 1999;80:615.
85. Robinson MH, Spruce L, Eeles R, et al. Limb function following conservation treatment of adult soft tissue sarcoma. Eur J Cancer 1991;27:1567.
86. Gerrand CH, Wunder JS, Kandel RA, et al. The influence of anatomic location on functional outcome in lower-extremity soft-tissue sarcoma. Ann Surg Oncol 2004;11:476.
87. Aksnes LH, Bauer HC, Jebsen NL, et al. Limb-sparing surgery preserves more function than amputation: a Scandinavian sarcoma group study of 118 patients. J Bone Joint Surg Br 2008;90:786.
88. Sugarbaker PH, Barofsky I, Rosenberg SA, et al. Quality of life assessment of patients in extremity sarcoma clinical trials. Surgery 1982;91:17.
89. Weddington WW Jr, Segraves KB, Simon MA. Psychological outcome of extremity sarcoma survivors undergoing amputation or limb salvage. J Clin Oncol 1985;3:1393.
90. Zagars GK, Ballo MT, Pisters PW, et al. Prognostic factors for patients with localized soft-tissue sarcoma treated with conservation surgery and radiation therapy: an analysis of 1225 patients. Cancer 2003;97:2530.
91. Catton C, Davis A, Bell R, et al. Soft tissue sarcoma of the extremity. Limb salvage after failure of combined conservative therapy. Radiother Oncol 1996; 41:209.
92. Karakousis CP, Proimakis C, Rao U, et al. Local recurrence and survival in soft-tissue sarcomas. Ann Surg Oncol 1996;3:255.

93. Ueda T, Yoshikawa H, Mori S, et al. Influence of local recurrence on the prognosis of soft-tissue sarcomas. J Bone Joint Surg Br 1997;79:553.

94. Pearlstone DB, Janjan NA, Feig BW, et al. Re-resection with brachytherapy for locally recurrent soft tissue sarcoma arising in a previously radiated field [see comments]. Cancer J Sci Am 1999;5:26.

95. Pickering DG, Stewart JS, Rampling R, et al. Fast neutron therapy for soft tissue sarcoma. Int J Radiat Oncol Biol Phys 1987;13:1489.

96. Schmitt G, Pape H, Zamboglou N. Long term results of neutron- and neutron-boost irradiation of soft tissue sarcomas. Strahlenther Onkol 1990;166:61.

97. Steingraber M, Lessel A, Jahn U. Fast neutron therapy in treatment of soft tissue sarcoma–the Berlin-Buch study. Bull Cancer Radiother 1996;83:122s.

98. Goffman T, Tochner Z, Glatstein E. Primary treatment of large and massive adult sarcomas with iododeoxyuridine and aggressive hyperfractionated irradiation. Cancer 1991;67:572.

99. Jakob J, Wenz F, Dinter DJ, et al. Preoperative intensity-modulated radiotherapy combined with temozolomide for locally advanced soft-tissue sarcoma. Int J Radiat Oncol Biol Phys 2009;75:810.

100. Rhomberg W, Hassenstein EO, Gefeller D. Radiotherapy vs. radiotherapy and razoxane in the treatment of soft tissue sarcomas: final results of a randomized study. Int J Radiat Oncol Biol Phys 1996;36:1077.

101. Blay JY, von Mehren M, Samuels BL, et al. Phase I combination study of trabectedin and doxorubicin in patients with soft-tissue sarcoma. Clin Cancer Res 2008;14:6656.

102. Garcia-Carbonero R, Supko JG, Maki RG, et al. Ecteinascidin-743 (ET-743) for chemotherapy-naive patients with advanced soft tissue sarcomas: multicenter phase II and pharmacokinetic study. J Clin Oncol 2005;23:5484.

103. Mendenhall WM, Zlotecki RA, Hochwald SN, et al. Retroperitoneal soft tissue sarcoma. Cancer 2005;104:669.

104. Pisters PW, O'Sullivan B. Retroperitoneal sarcomas: combined modality treatment approaches. Curr Opin Oncol 2002;14:400.

105. Lewis JJ, Leung D, Woodruff JM, et al. Retroperitoneal soft-tissue sarcoma: analysis of 500 patients treated and followed at a single institution. Ann Surg 1998;228:355.

106. Stoeckle E, Coindre JM, Bonvalot S, et al. Prognostic factors in retroperitoneal sarcoma: a multivariate analysis of a series of 165 patients of the French Cancer Center Federation Sarcoma Group. Cancer 2001;92:359.

107. Singer S, Antonescu CR, Riedel E, et al. Histologic subtype and margin of resection predict pattern of recurrence and survival for retroperitoneal liposarcoma. Ann Surg 2003;238:358.

108. van Dalen T, Hoekstra HJ, van Geel AN, et al. Locoregional recurrence of retroperitoneal soft tissue sarcoma: second chance of cure for selected patients. Eur J Surg Oncol 2001;27:564.

109. Russo P, Kim Y, Ravindran S, et al. Nephrectomy during operative management of retroperitoneal sarcoma. Ann Surg Oncol 1997;4:421.

110. Petersen IA, Haddock MG, Donohue JH, et al. Use of intraoperative electron beam radiotherapy in the management of retroperitoneal soft tissue sarcomas. Int J Radiat Oncol Biol Phys 2002;52:469.

111. Jones JJ, Catton CN, O'Sullivan B, et al. Initial results of a trial of preoperative external-beam radiation therapy and postoperative brachytherapy for retroperitoneal sarcoma. Ann Surg Oncol 2002;9:346.

112. Gieschen HL, Spiro IJ, Suit HD, et al. Long-term results of intraoperative electron beam radiotherapy for primary and recurrent retroperitoneal soft tissue sarcoma. Int J Radiat Oncol Biol Phys 2001;50:127.

113. Eilber FC, Rosen G, Nelson SD, et al. High-grade extremity soft tissue sarcomas: factors predictive of local recurrence and its effect on morbidity and mortality. Ann Surg 2003;237:218.

114. Tanabe KK, Pollock RE, Ellis LM, et al. Influence of surgical margins on outcome in patients with preoperatively irradiated extremity soft tissue sarcomas. Cancer 1994;73:1652.

115. Robertson JM, Sondak VK, Weiss SA, et al. Preoperative radiation therapy and iododeoxyuridine for large retroperitoneal sarcomas. Int J Radiat Oncol Biol Phys 1995;31:87.

Adjuvant Chemotherapy for Soft Tissue Sarcomas

Vinod Ravi, MD*, Shreyaskumar Patel, MD

KEYWORDS

- Soft tissue sarcomas • Adjuvant chemotherapy
- Neoadjuvant chemotherapy • Mesenchymal neoplasms

Soft tissue sarcomas (STS) are mesenchymal neoplasms arising from the connective tissue in the body. There is considerable heterogeneity among STS with more than 50 distinct histologic subtypes. Each of these histologic subtypes represents a unique disease with distinct biologic behavior and varying sensitivity to chemotherapy. Approximately 54% of STS are localized at diagnosis,[1] representing a potentially curable subpopulation. Four thousand patients die of STS every year,[2] mostly from distant metastatic disease. The judicious use of adjuvant/neoadjuvant chemotherapy along with surgery and radiation in the treatment of localized STS has a role in improving patient outcomes by decreasing local and distant recurrences.[3]

The use of adjuvant chemotherapy in an unselected population results in limited benefit.[4] In the authors' opinion, it is important to identify the subpopulation that is most likely to die of metastatic disease. The application of effective therapies in this subset will result in the most benefit. There are 2 prerequisites to effective adjuvant therapy: (1) the identification of patients who are high risk for developing fatal metastatic disease and (2) the availability of effective histology-specific treatment options. For example, adjuvant therapy for rhabdomyosarcoma, a biologically aggressive histologic subtype with high metastatic potential, using effective treatment regimens results in significant clinical benefit.[5] A primary tumor size greater than 5 cm, high grade, tumor involving or deep to the fascia, specific histologic subtypes (**Table 1**), and recurrent disease are all associated with a higher likelihood of developing metastatic disease.[6,7]

Most patients with distant relapse tend to die of their disease,[3] so early incorporation of adjuvant chemotherapy in the multidisciplinary treatment to eradicate micrometastases is important. Combination regimens used extensively in the treatment of STS include (1) Adriamycin/ifosfamide, (2) Adriamycin/dacarbazine, and (3) gemcitabine/ docetaxel. However, the sensitivity of various subtypes to these combinations is

Department of Sarcoma Medical Oncology, University of Texas MD Anderson Cancer Center, 1515 Holcombe Boulevard, Unit 450, Houston, TX 77030, USA
* Corresponding author.
E-mail address: vravi@mdanderson.org

Table 1
The metastatic potential for various histologic subtypes of soft tissue sarcoma

Low Metastatic Potential	Intermediate Metastatic Potential	High Metastatic Potential
Well-differentiated liposarcoma	Inflammatory myofibroblastic tumor	Pleomorphic liposarcoma
	Epithelioid hemangioendothelioma	Dedifferentiated liposarcoma
	Solitary fibrous tumor Hemangiopericytoma	Leiomyosarcoma
		Round cell liposarcoma
		Malignant fibrous histiocytoma
		Angiosarcoma
		Rhabdomyosarcoma
		Synovial sarcoma
		Extraskeletal Ewing sarcoma
		Epithelioid sarcoma
		Alveolar soft parts sarcoma
		Gastrointestinal stromal tumor

different and should be taken into account. For example, some STS, such as alveolar soft part sarcoma (ASPS), have a high propensity for metastases but with minimally effective systemic therapy options. Consequently, ASPS should be treated with local therapy; adjuvant systemic therapy should be avoided outside of a clinical trial.

ADJUVANT SYSTEMIC CHEMOTHERAPY FOR STS
Prospective Studies of Adriamycin

Adriamycin was introduced as an active agent for advanced STS in the 1970s.[8,9] One of the earliest randomized clinical trials examining the role of adjuvant chemotherapy was done at the National Cancer Institute where Dr Rosenberg and colleagues[10] randomized 65 patients with high-grade extremity STS to receive either adjuvant Adriamycin, cyclophosphamide, and methotrexate or no chemotherapy. They were able to demonstrate improved disease-free survival (DFS) and overall survival (OS) in the adjuvant chemotherapy group (3 years DFS 92% vs 60%, OS 95% vs 74%). There was no local recurrence (LR) in the adjuvant therapy group as compared with 2 LR in the no chemotherapy group. Interestingly, synovial sarcoma and rhabdomyosarcoma, 2 histologic subtypes with aggressive biologic behavior, were disproportionately more prevalent in the adjuvant therapy group. This imbalance did not adversely affect the outcome of the chemotherapy group, supporting the hypothesis that the benefit of adjuvant chemotherapy is best demonstrated in aggressive STS subtypes.

Similarly, Gherlinzoni and colleagues[11] randomized 59 high-grade STS to receive either Adriamycin 450 mg/m^2 or no adjuvant therapy after surgery and radiation. DFS in the adjuvant chemotherapy group was 79.1% versus 54.3% in the no chemotherapy group. Development of pulmonary metastases was much more frequent in the no chemotherapy group (40%) as compared with the adjuvant chemotherapy group (16.6%). LR was also more common in the no chemotherapy group (8.6% vs 4.1%).

Antman and colleagues[12] randomized 42 patients to receive 5 cycles of adjuvant Adriamycin 90 mg/m^2 every 3 weeks versus observation. The largest histologic subtype enrolled was liposarcoma (40% in the treatment group and 32% in the observation group), but this histology was not further subclassified into well-differentiated, dedifferentiated, pleomorphic, or myxoid subtypes. Besides liposarcoma, the trial enrolled 9 other histologic types of STS. The authors reported a 12% improvement in DFS and an 8% improvement in OS for adjuvant chemotherapy. However, this failed to achieve statistical significance because of the small sample size.

Prospective Studies of Adriamycin and Ifosfamide

Brodowicz and colleagues[13] randomized 59 patients to receive 6 courses of adjuvant Adriamycin (50 mg/m^2 per cycle), ifosfamide (6 g/m^2 per cycle), and dacarbazine (800 mg/m^2 per cycle) versus observation after the resection of localized STS. Grade 3 tumors were present in 81% of patients in the chemotherapy arm and 57% of patients in the control arm. Despite higher preponderance of high grade within the chemotherapy arm, 77% of patients in this group were recurrence free versus 57% of patients in the control arm (mean follow-up 41 months). The relapse-free survival, time to local failure, time to distant failure, and OS were not significantly different between the 2 treatment groups, likely because of the small sample size and short follow-up.

Frustaci and colleagues[14] randomized 104 patients with high-grade extremity STS greater than or equal to 5 cm to receive 5 cycles of epirubicin (120 mg/m^2 per cycle) and ifosfamide (9 g/m^2 per cycle) or observation after local therapy. At a median follow-up of 59 months, median DFS was 48 months in the treatment group versus 16 months in the control group. The median OS was 75 months for the treatment group as compared with 46 months for the control group. For OS, the absolute benefit from chemotherapy was 13% at 2 years and increased to 19% at 4 years (**Table 2**). The authors published follow-up data 2 years later showing a 5-year OS of 66% versus 46% favoring adjuvant therapy ($P = .04$). However, longer follow-up after 89.6 months showed that the difference favoring adjuvant therapy lost statistical significance ($P = .07$).[15]

Petrioli and colleagues[16] randomized 88 patients with high-risk STS to receive chemotherapy versus observation. Of the 45 patients enrolled into the chemotherapy arm, 26 patients received epirubicin and 19 patients received epirubicin and ifosfamide. Fifty-two percent were in an extremity location, and 41% were high grade. Unfortunately, the trial closed early because of poor accrual. At a median follow-up of 94 months, the relapse rate was 29% in the adjuvant arm versus 46% in the control arm ($P = .1$). There was a statistically significant difference in the estimated 5-year DFS between the adjuvant arm (69%) and control arm (44%) ($P = .01$). Five-year OS for patients who received adjuvant therapy was 72% versus 47% in the control arm. However, the difference was not statistically significant ($P = .06$). Because this trial contained an anthracycline-only subgroup and an anthracycline and ifosfamide subgroup, review of the results of the subgroup analysis would be of interest to determine the role, if any, of the addition of ifosfamide to anthracyclines, which has been debated over time. There was a statistically significant difference in the estimated the 5-year DFS between the epirubicin and ifosfamide subgroup and the control group, whereas the difference between the epirubicin-only subgroup and the control group was not statistically significant. Similarly, the 5-year DFS for the epirubicin and ifosfamide subgroup compared with the control was significantly better (84% vs 57%, $P = .01$). The number of patients in the epirubicin and ifosfamide subset is much less than for the epirubicin-only subset. Despite this, the smaller subset (epirubicin and ifosfamide) continues to retain statistical significance, suggesting a role for the addition of ifosfamide to anthracyclines as an adjuvant therapy for high-risk STS.

Along similar lines, Eilber and colleagues[17] demonstrated that the addition of ifosfamide to Adriamycin and cisplatin (along with radiation) resulted in greater than or equal to 95% pathologic necrosis in 48% of patients (n = 81) compared with 13% in other

Table 2
Clinical trials examining the role of adjuvant chemotherapy for soft tissue sarcomas

Year	Author	Patients	Histologic Subtypes[a]	High Grade (%)	Site	Regimen/Dose	Measure	Outcome Rx (%)	Control (%)	Statistical Significance
1983	Rosenberg et al[10]	65	MFH, Synovial sarcoma, Liposarcoma	78	E	ADM 50–70 mg/m²[b], CTX 500–700 mg/m², MTX 50–250 mg/kg[c]	DFS at 3 y, OS, LR	92, 95, 0	60, 74, 7	S, S
1984	Antman et al[12]	42	Liposarcoma mixed[d]	74	E, T	ADM 90 mg/m²	DFS, OS	80, 85	68, 77	NS, NS
1986	Gherlinzoni et al[11]	59	MFH, Synovial sarcoma, Fibrosarcoma	100	E	ADM 450 mg/m² (cumulative)	DFS, Lung mets, LR	79, 17, 4	54, 40, 9	S
2000	Brodowicz et al[13]	59	Liposarcoma, MFH, Synovial sarcoma	69	E, T	ADM 50 mg/m², IF 6 g/m², DTIC 800 mg/m²	DFS, LR, DR	77, 6, 19	57, 21, 36	NS, NS, NS
2001	Frustaci et al[14]	104	MFH, Synovial sarcoma, Liposarcoma	100	E	EPI 120 mg/m², IF 9 g/m²	DFS 2 y, DFS 4 y, LR 2 y[e], LR 4 y[e], DR 2 y[e], DR 4 y[e], OS 2 y, OS 4 y	72, 50, 0, 6, 28, 44, 85, 69	45, 37, 10, 17, 45, 45, 72, 50	S, NS, S, NS, NS, NS, NS, S

Year	Reference	N	Histology		ADJ	Dose	Outcome			Significance
2002	Petrioli et al[16]	88	MFH Liposarcoma Leiomyosarcoma	41	E, T	EPI 75 mg/m² IF 6 g/m²	DFS 5 y OS 5 y	69 72	44 47	S NS
2007[f]	Woll PJ et al[18]	351	Leiomyosarcoma Liposarcoma MFH Synovial sarcoma[g]	60	E, T	ADM 75 mg/m² IF 5 g/m²	DFS 5 y OS	52 64	52 69	NS NS

Abbreviations: ActD, actinomycin D; ADJ, adjuvant therapy group; ADM, Adriamycin; CTX, cyclophosphamide; DFS, disease-free survival; DR, distant recurrence; DTIC, dacarbazine; E, extremity; EPI, epirubicin; IF, ifosfamide; LR, local recurrence; mets, metastases; MFH, malignant fibrous histiocytoma; MTX, methotrexate; NS, difference is not statistically significant; S, statistically significant difference; T, trunk; VCR, vincristine.

a For clinical trials that enrolled multiple histologic subtypes, the 3 most common histologic subtypes are listed here.
b Cumulative ADM dose less than 550 mg/m² in all patients.
c MTX administered after cumulative ADM dose of 550 mg/m² reached.
d Nine different sarcomas subtypes.
e Cumulative incidence.
f Study has not been published. Presented at the 2007 Annual American Society of Clinical Oncology meeting.
g Both MFH and synovial sarcoma had equal prevalence in the study population based on published abstract.

Adriamycin-containing regimens (including Adriamycin and cisplatin). This finding also resulted in statistically significant improvements in 5-year and 10-year survival (77% and 71%, respectively).

The interim analysis of the most recent and the largest European Organisation for Research and Treatment of Cancer (EORTC) adjuvant chemotherapy trial[18] in patients with intermediate and high-grade STS (presented at the 2007 American Society of Clinical Oncology [ASCO] annual meeting by Woll and colleagues[18]) showed no benefit to adjuvant chemotherapy. The results of this trial have not been published, making it difficult to analyze the results. However, it is important to note that this trial enrolled patients with intermediate-grade tumors (40% of the study population) and used a lower dose of ifosfamide at $5gm/m^2$. The lack of benefit may be a function of suboptimal chemotherapy and a poorly selected, heterogeneous population of patients.

Meta-Analysis of Adjuvant Chemotherapy Trials

For a rare disease, clinical trials are often plagued by a small number of participants, limiting the trial's ability to detect small differences between the study groups. The Sarcoma Meta-Analysis Collaboration (SMAC) chose to address this problem by combining small, individual clinical trials with few patients into a large meta-analysis that would be adequately powered to reliably detect a moderate treatment effect. Tierney and colleagues[19] had previously reviewed 15 clinical trials to perform a meta-analysis of the published data, suggesting an improvement in OS in favor of adjuvant chemotherapy for extremity STS. Based on these findings, the SMAC[20] collected individual data on all randomized patients from eligible trials for an intention-to-treat analysis. The purpose of such an analysis was to identify if adjuvant chemotherapy improved survival in patients with localized STS, to quantify any effect of chemotherapy on the rates of local and distant recurrence, and to investigate whether certain groups of patients derive a greater benefit from chemotherapy. The meta-analysis included 14 trials totaling 1568 patients with a median follow-up of 9.4 years. Sixty-seven percent of the patients had high-grade tumors, and less than 5% were low grade. Only 9% of the patients had a liposarcoma. Other histologic subtypes included malignant fibrous histiocytoma (20%), leiomyosarcoma (12%), synovial sarcoma (10%), and other sarcomas (31%). The total cumulative dose of Adriamycin administered ranged from 200 to 550 mg/m^2, with a dose per cycle of 50 to 90 mg/m^2. Patients in the chemotherapy arm were noted to have a 27% reduction in the risk for LR and a 30% reduction in the risk of metastases (absolute benefit of 10% was sustained at 10 years). There was a trend toward improved OS with chemotherapy with an 11% risk reduction (4% sustained at 10 years), but this was not statistically significant.

In 2008, Pervaiz and colleagues[21] included 4 additional randomized control trials (RCTs) published since the original SMAC publication into a meta-analysis of 18 RCTs. Five out of the 18 RCTs used Adriamycin combined with ifosfamide. In these trials, the Adriamycin dosage ranged from 50 to 90 mg/m^2 per cycle and the ifosfamide dosage ranged from 1500 to 5000 mg/m^2 per cycle. The updated meta-analysis showed a statistically significant reduction in both local and distant recurrences and a better OS for patients receiving chemotherapy as compared with observation. The addition of Adriamycin and ifosfamide–containing RCTs showed a trend toward a further reduction in recurrence risk and increased survival as compared with Adriamycin alone.

NEOADJUVANT CHEMOTHERAPY FOR STS

As previously described, several prospective studies have suggested a beneficial role for adjuvant systemic chemotherapy (see **Table 2**). The marked heterogeneity of the study populations in these trials, along with small sample sizes, makes it difficult to extrapolate these results to an individual sarcoma patient with a specific histopathologic diagnosis. Moreover, even within specific histopathologic subtypes, the response to chemotherapy can be variable. The modest benefit demonstrated by many of the clinical trials listed in **Table 2** may be the result of the dilution of the small but real benefit for some patients by the larger number of nonresponders. Neoadjuvant therapy presents an attractive opportunity to weed out the nonresponders from the responders because of its ability to function as an in vivo drug trial by assessing the primary tumor response.

Neoadjuvant chemotherapy requires effective imaging tools to identify a response to treatment. In an attempt to determine the utility of functional imaging techniques in the neoadjuvant setting, Scheutze and colleagues[22] evaluated 46 patients with high-grade localized STS using (F-18)-fluorodeoxyglucose (FDG) positron emission tomography (PET) before and after neoadjuvant chemotherapy. All patients received Adriamycin-containing combination chemotherapy. Patients received 2 to 4 cycles of neoadjuvant chemotherapy, with most receiving 3 cycles before surgery. Including neoadjuvant and adjuvant, the median number of total chemotherapy cycles was 7. At a median follow-up of 46 months, 52% of the patients remained recurrence free, 39% developed metastatic disease, and 9% developed an LR recurrence as a first event. An maximum standardized uptake value (SUVmax) greater than or equal to 6 at baseline was a statistically significant predictor of metastases. Patients with a greater than or equal to 40% decrease in SUVmax had a significantly lower risk of disease recurrence and metastases. These patients also had a statistically significant improvement in OS. No differences were noted between changes in SUVmax after 2 versus 3 versus 4 cycles of preoperative therapy. Therefore, PET/computed tomography may be a valuable tool in the early assessment of the response to chemotherapy because the change in SUVmax correlates with the disease recurrence risk.

Gortzak and colleagues[23] used a combination of Adriamycin and ifosfamide (Adriamycin 50 mg/m^2, ifosfamide 5 g/m^2 for only 3 cycles) in the neoadjuvant setting for high-risk STS and failed to demonstrate any DFS or OS advantage. As previously discussed, Eilber and colleagues[17] evaluated the role of multi-agent chemotherapy combined with radiation in the neoadjuvant setting and found greater percent necrosis, improved survival, and a decreased rate of LR in patients receiving an ifosfamide-containing regimen.[22] There was also a statistically significant decrease in LR rates and an improved survival for patients with greater than or equal to 95% pathologic necrosis.

HISTOLOGY-SPECIFIC ADJUVANT CHEMOTHERAPY TRIALS

Heterogeneity within the study population has been postulated as one of the reasons why clinical trials evaluating adjuvant therapy among high-risk STS have failed to show statistically significant outcomes, even though the trend toward benefit is almost always present. Specific histologic subtypes that do not respond well to chemotherapy when mixed in with chemosensitive subtypes may attenuate the true benefit in the sensitive subtypes. Prospective studies examining adjuvant chemotherapy in specific STS histologic subtypes (to ensure a homogenous study population) are reviewed later.

Synovial Sarcoma

Eilber and colleagues[24] prospectively collected data on 101 patients with synovial sarcoma who underwent surgical treatment with curative intent from 1992 to 2002.

Sixty-seven percent of the patients were treated with ifosfamide-based therapy (2 patients received Adriamycin-based chemotherapy that did not contain ifosfamide) and 33% received no chemotherapy. Among patients who received ifosfamide-based therapy, 85% had neoadjuvant therapy (and all patients received Adriamycin). At a median follow-up of 58 months, patients treated with ifosfamide-based therapy (in combination with Adriamycin) had a 2-year disease-specific survival (DSS) of 96% versus 87% for patients who received no chemotherapy. At 4 years, DSS for ifosfamide-treated patients was 88% compared with 67% in the no-chemotherapy patients. Ifosfamide-based chemotherapy emerged as an important independent predictor for survival in a multivariate model. Similarly, the 4-year recurrence-free survival for patients treated with ifosfamide-based therapy was 74% versus 46% for patients who received no chemotherapy. Their conclusion was that, for patients with synovial sarcoma, chemotherapy with a combination of ifosfamide and Adriamycin is associated with significant benefit for both recurrence and survival endpoints.

Liposarcoma

Eliber and colleagues[25] reported on 245 patients with extremity liposarcoma undergoing potentially curative surgery; 26% were treated with ifosfamide-based chemotherapy, 34% with Adriamycin-based chemotherapy, and 40% did not receive chemotherapy. The 5-year DSS for the ifosfamide-treated patients was 92% as compared with 65% for the no-chemotherapy patients. This difference was statistically significant. Therefore, ifosfamide (in combination with Adriamycin) should be strongly considered for the treatment of patients with extremity liposarcoma.

Leiomyosarcoma

Hensley and colleagues[26] examined the use of adjuvant gemcitabine plus docetaxel for 25 patients with completely resected high-grade stage I to IV uterine leiomyosarcoma. Gemcitabine was dosed at 900 mg/m^2 on day 1 and day 8, with docetaxel at 75 mg/m^2 on day 8 of a 21-day cycle. At a median follow-up of 49 months, the 2-year progression-free survival (PFS) was 45% (a median PFS of 13 months). Among patients with stage I to II uterine leiomyosarcoma, the 2-year PFS was 59% (a median PFS of 39 months). Based on historical data, patients with leiomyosarcoma who undergo complete resection have a 2-year recurrence rate of 50% to 80%.[26] Therefore, adjuvant gemcitabine and docetaxel seem to decrease the potential for recurrence. The only randomized trial evaluating the role of adjuvant Adriamycin in uterine leiomyosarcoma was reported by Omura and colleagues.[27] The156 patients wit uterine sarcomas included 48 cases of leiomyosarcoma. In the leiomyosarcoma subset, 44% of the patients who received Adriamycin at 60 mg/m^2 (8 cycles) recurred, whereas 61% of the patients in the observation arm recurred. Unfortunately, the presence of multiple histologic subtypes in the trial limited the interpretation. Based on the previously mentioned findings, Hensley and colleagues[28] conducted a multi-institutional adjuvant therapy phase II trial combining 4 cycles of gemcitabine/docetaxel with 4 cycles of Adriamycin in 47 women with completely resected uterine leiomyosarcoma. At a median follow-up of 23 months, 78% of the women remained progression free. These findings are still preliminary and will require longer follow-up.

Bone Sarcomas

Osteosarcoma and Ewing sarcoma represent 2 excellent examples of the beneficial role of chemotherapy in the treatment of sarcomas with high metastatic potential. There is a statistically significant improvement in both DFS and OS using adjuvant therapy in these histologic subtypes.[29–32] Both osteosarcoma and Ewing sarcoma tend to metastasize early, and neoadjuvant therapy followed by surgery followed by adjuvant therapy has become the standard of care. Neoadjuvant therapy allows for the evaluation of the response to chemotherapy and can be an effective prognostic tool that helps in the selection of drugs for more optimal adjuvant therapy. Patients with a poor pathologic response to neoadjuvant therapy tend to have a high probability of developing metastatic disease and dying of their sarcoma.[33,34]

Gastrointestinal Stromal Tumors

As discussed in the gastrointestinal stromal tumors (GIST) article of this issue, the benefit of adjuvant therapy may not be limited to cytotoxic chemotherapy. Targeted agents, such as imatinib, can have an equally significant impact. The American College of Surgeons Oncology Group (ACOSOG) Z9001 trial established the benefit of adjuvant imatinib 400 mg daily over placebo in completely resected GIST at least 3 cm in size. At a median follow-up of 20 months, the trial was stopped early because of a higher number of recurrences in the placebo group. The 1-year, relapse-free survival was 98% versus 83%, favoring imatinib (hazard ratio 0.35).

THE CONTROVERSY AND SUMMARY

Except for a few trials that have shown a statistically significant improvement in DFS[10,11,14] and OS,[10,14] most of the STS adjuvant therapy clinical trials done in the last 20 years have only shown a trend toward improved survival (see **Table 2**). Even in trials that have shown a significant survival difference, some have not retained their statistical significance on follow-up past 5 years.[15] Interim analysis of the most recent and largest EORTC adjuvant chemotherapy trial[18] that enrolled 351 patients (presented at the 2007 ASCO annual meeting) failed to show any benefit from adjuvant therapy. Consequently, many clinicians have concluded that there is no benefit to adjuvant chemotherapy in STS.[4]

Based on the data outlined in the previous sections, the authors would argue that the lack of benefit might be related to a heterogeneous patient population, inadequate chemotherapy, and poor patient selection (including intermediate grade tumors that are less likely to respond to chemotherapy). Clinical trials that have enrolled homogenous patient populations (eg, limited to one histology) at high risk for developing metastatic disease (eg, >5 cm, high grade) and have used histology specific, effective treatment regimens have shown significant benefits. GIST, rhabdomyosarcoma, Ewing sarcoma, and osteosarcoma are excellent examples whereby a specific histologic subtype treated with chemotherapy tailored to the disease can produce survival advantages that are sustained over time. Therefore, the authors think that, in well-selected, high-risk patients, adjuvant chemotherapy (or preferably neoadjuvant therapy) using agents known to be active in that histologic subtype can have a significant clinical benefit.

In high-risk STS histologic subtypes known to have only a modest response to chemotherapy, neoadjuvant therapy with close monitoring of the response is recommended. Neoadjuvant therapy can act as an in vivo assessment to determine the sensitivity of an individual tumor. This finding has both prognostic significance and clinical utility for planning additional adjuvant systemic therapy. Neoadjuvant therapy also limits unnecessary ongoing chemotherapy toxicity in a poor responder. Finally, the use of novel imaging techniques, such as functional imaging (FDG-PET), during neoadjuvant therapy may help predict which patients are likely to derive the most benefit. Future trials examining the role of adjuvant therapy should consider a neoadjuvant component with early functional imaging to identify patients who are likely to benefit and to limit toxicity in the nonresponders.

REFERENCES

1. SEER stat fact sheets: soft tissue including heart. National Cancer Institute; 2011. Available at: http://seer.cancer.gov/statfacts/html/soft.html. Accessed November 2, 2011.
2. United States Cancer Statistics: 1999–2007 incidence and mortality web-based report. U.S. Department of Health and Human Services, Centers for Disease Control and Prevention and National Cancer Institute. Available at: http://www.cdc.gov/uscs. Accessed November 19, 2011.
3. Schuetze SM, Patel S. Should patients with high-risk soft tissue sarcoma receive adjuvant chemotherapy? Oncologist 2009;14:1003–12.
4. Blay JY, Le Cesne A. Adjuvant chemotherapy in localized soft tissue sarcomas: still not proven. Oncologist 2009;14:1013–20. [Epub Oct 6 2009].
5. Ferrer FA, Isakoff M, Koyle MA. Bladder/prostate rhabdomyosarcoma: past, present and future. J Urol 2006;176:1283–91.
6. Pisters PW, Leung DH, Woodruff J, et al. Analysis of prognostic factors in 1,041 patients with localized soft tissue sarcomas of the extremities. J Clin Oncol 1996; 14:1679–89.
7. Weitz J, Antonescu CR, Brennan MF. Localized extremity soft tissue sarcoma: improved knowledge with unchanged survival over time. J Clin Oncol 2003;21: 2719–25.
8. Benjamin RS, Wiernik PH, Bachur NR. Adriamycin: a new effective agent in the therapy of disseminated sarcomas. Med Pediatr Oncol 1975;1:63–76.
9. O'Bryan RM, Luce JK, Talley RW, et al. Phase II evaluation of Adriamycin in human neoplasia. Cancer 1973;32:1–8.
10. Rosenberg SA, Tepper J, Glatstein E, et al. Prospective randomized evaluation of adjuvant chemotherapy in adults with soft tissue sarcomas of the extremities. Cancer 1983;52:424–34.
11. Gherlinzoni F, Bacci G, Picci P, et al. A randomized trial for the treatment of high-grade soft-tissue sarcomas of the extremities: preliminary observations. J Clin Oncol 1986;4:552–8.
12. Antman K, Suit H, Amato D, et al. Preliminary results of a randomized trial of adjuvant doxorubicin for sarcomas: lack of apparent difference between treatment groups. J Clin Oncol 1984;2:601–8.
13. Brodowicz T, Schwameis E, Widder J, et al. Intensified adjuvant IFADIC chemotherapy for adult soft tissue sarcoma: a prospective randomized feasibility trial. Sarcoma 2000;4:151–60.
14. Frustaci S, Gherlinzoni F, De Paoli A, et al. Adjuvant chemotherapy for adult soft tissue sarcomas of the extremities and girdles: results of the Italian randomized cooperative trial. J Clin Oncol 2001;19:1238–47.
15. Frustaci S, De Paoli A, Bidoli E, et al. Ifosfamide in the adjuvant therapy of soft tissue sarcomas. Oncology 2003;65:80–4.
16. Petrioli R, Coratti A, Correale P, et al. Adjuvant epirubicin with or without ifosfamide for adult soft-tissue sarcoma. Am J Clin Oncol 2002;25:468–73.
17. Eilber FC, Rosen G, Eckardt J, et al. Treatment-induced pathologic necrosis: a predictor of local recurrence and survival in patients receiving neoadjuvant therapy for high-grade extremity soft tissue sarcomas. J Clin Oncol 2001;19: 3203–9.
18. Woll PJ, van Glabbeke M, Hohenberger P, et al. Adjuvant chemotherapy (CT) with doxorubicin and ifosfamide in resected soft tissue sarcoma (STS): interim analysis of a randomised phase III trial. J Clin Oncol 2007;10008.

19. Tierney JF, Mosseri V, Stewart LA, et al. Adjuvant chemotherapy for soft-tissue sarcoma: review and meta-analysis of the published results of randomised clinical trials. Br J Cancer 1995;72:469–75.
20. Adjuvant chemotherapy for localised resectable soft-tissue sarcoma of adults: meta-analysis of individual data. Sarcoma Meta-analysis Collaboration. Lancet 1997;350:1647–54.
21. Pervaiz N, Colterjohn N, Farrokhyar F, et al. A systematic meta-analysis of randomized controlled trials of adjuvant chemotherapy for localized resectable soft-tissue sarcoma. Cancer 2008;113:573–81.
22. Schuetze SM, Rubin BP, Vernon C, et al. Use of positron emission tomography in localized extremity soft tissue sarcoma treated with neoadjuvant chemotherapy. Cancer 2005;103:339–48.
23. Gortzak E, Azzarelli A, Buesa J, et al. A randomised phase II study on neoadjuvant chemotherapy for 'high-risk' adult soft-tissue sarcoma. Eur J Cancer 2001;37:1096–103.
24. Eilber FC, Brennan MF, Eilber FR, et al. Chemotherapy is associated with improved survival in adult patients with primary extremity synovial sarcoma. Ann Surg 2007;246:105–13.
25. Eilber FC, Eilber FR, Eckardt J, et al. The impact of chemotherapy on the survival of patients with high-grade primary extremity liposarcoma. Ann Surg 2004;240:686–95 [discussion: 95–7].
26. Hensley ML, Ishill N, Soslow R, et al. Adjuvant gemcitabine plus docetaxel for completely resected stages I–IV high grade uterine leiomyosarcoma: results of a prospective study. Gynecol Oncol 2009;112:563–7.
27. Omura GA, Blessing JA, Major F, et al. A randomized clinical trial of adjuvant Adriamycin in uterine sarcomas: a Gynecologic Oncology Group study. J Clin Oncol 1985;3:1240–5.
28. Hensley ML, Wathen K, Maki RG, et al. Adjuvant treatment of high-risk primary uterine leiomyosarcoma with gemcitabine/docetaxel (GT), followed by doxorubicin (D): results of phase II multicenter trial SARC005. In: 2010 ASCO Annual Meeting. Chicago (IL), 2010: J Clin Oncol Author Anonymous [Suppl; abstract: 10021] 2010;28:15s.
29. Eilber F, Giuliano A, Eckardt J, et al. Adjuvant chemotherapy for osteosarcoma: a randomized prospective trial. J Clin Oncol 1987;5:21–6.
30. Grier HE, Krailo MD, Tarbell NJ, et al. Addition of ifosfamide and etoposide to standard chemotherapy for Ewing's sarcoma and primitive neuroectodermal tumor of bone. N Engl J Med 2003;348:694–701.
31. Link MP, Goorin AM, Miser AW, et al. The effect of adjuvant chemotherapy on relapse-free survival in patients with osteosarcoma of the extremity. N Engl J Med 1986;314:1600–6.
32. Nesbit ME Jr, Gehan EA, Burgert EO Jr, et al. Multimodal therapy for the management of primary, nonmetastatic Ewing's sarcoma of bone: a long-term follow-up of the first intergroup study. J Clin Oncol 1990;8:1664–74.
33. Wunder JS, Paulian G, Huvos AG, et al. The histological response to chemotherapy as a predictor of the oncological outcome of operative treatment of Ewing sarcoma. J Bone Joint Surg Am 1998;80:1020–33.
34. Bacci G, Bertoni F, Longhi A, et al. Neoadjuvant chemotherapy for high-grade central osteosarcoma of the extremity. Histologic response to preoperative chemotherapy correlates with histologic subtype of the tumor. Cancer 2003;97:3068–75.

Margin Status, Local Recurrence, and Survival: Correlation or Causation?

Steven J. Nurkin, MD[a], John M. Kane III, MD[a,b],*

KEYWORDS

- Sarcoma • Margin status • Sarcoma recurrence and survival

There is an inherent complexity to managing patients with soft tissue sarcomas (STS). They are comparatively rare tumors with multiple histologies and anatomic variability. STS may also have unpredictable biologic behavior that can lead to late recurrence or distant metastases. Important variables that influence STS outcomes are divided into 3 main categories. First are patient factors that include age, sex, the anatomic location of the primary tumor, and depth. Second, and probably the most important, are tumor factors such as size, grade, and the specific histology. Third are treatment factors that include the adequacy of the surgical resection and the effect of adjuvant therapies. There is an interaction between all of these prognostic factors. Studies have shown that large, deep, high-grade STS at certain locations (such as head and neck or retroperitoneum) have a significantly increased risk for a positive-margin surgical resection.[1] But the critical question is whether this is caused by bad surgery, a controllable variable, or bad biology, which cannot be controlled. Currently, the complex interaction between STS resection margin status, local recurrence (LR), and survival is not clear.

In 1982, Dr Rosenberg and the National Cancer Institute published a seminal paper that changed the surgical treatment of extremity STS.[2] This was a prospective study in which 43 patients with high-grade tumors were randomized to limb-sparing surgery plus radiation therapy (RT) versus amputation (both groups received systemic chemotherapy). The LR rate for the limb salvage group was 15% (1 successfully salvaged with amputation) compared with no LR in the amputation group ($P = .06$). However, there were no differences in 5-year disease-free survival (DFS) (71% vs 78%, $P = .75$) or overall survival (OS) (83% vs 88%; $P = .99$). A multivariate analysis of patients with

---

There was no funding to support this review, and the authors have nothing to disclose.
[a] Surgical Oncology, Roswell Park Cancer Institute, Elm and Carlton Streets, Buffalo, NY 14263, USA
[b] Department of Surgery, University of Buffalo, Buffalo, NY, USA
* Corresponding author. Roswell Park Cancer Institute, Elm and Carlton Streets, Buffalo, NY 14263.
E-mail address: John.Kane@roswellpark.org

STS from this study and another National Cancer Institute protocol showed that a positive resection margin was significantly associated with an increased risk for LR ($P<.0001$). The investigators had several provocative conclusions. First, an increased rate of LR did not seem to affect survival. Perhaps patients with an LR were simply more likely to develop distant metastases even if local control had been obtained with an amputation. In addition, if a negative-margin limb-sparing surgery could be combined with adjuvant radiation and chemotherapy, then long-term survival seemed to be comparable with amputation. Shortly thereafter, the National Institutes of Health formulated a consensus statement recommending limb-sparing surgery for most patients with high-grade extremity STS.[3]

WHAT IS THE APPROPRIATE STS RESECTION MARGIN?

Once limb-sparing surgery became the standard of care, the appropriate STS resection margin needed to be defined. Enneking[4] and others previously classified margins based on the type of surgical resection performed. With intralesional excision, the plane of excision has passed through the tumor, leaving microscopic or macroscopic tumor behind. With marginal excision, the gross tumor is removed within or close to the pseudocapsule with no attempt to remove a cuff of normal tissue. With wide excision, the gross tumor is removed with a rim of normal surrounding tissue. With compartmental (radical) excision, the entire compartment in which a tumor is located is removed. Retrospective studies of STS prognostic factors have correlated this classification with outcome.[5–7] LR after intralesional and marginal excisions has been unacceptably high.[6,8,9] In contrast, compartmental/radical excision, similar to amputation, has lower LR rates but at the expense of poorer limb function and decreased quality of life.[8]

In the modern limb salvage era, the optimal STS resection margin has generically been defined as the amount of tissue necessary to obtain a negative-margin resection.[10] In practice, this is typically at least 1 to 2 cm of grossly normal tissue around the tumor and the pseudocapsule (or less if there is an intact biologic tissue barrier such as fascia). However, especially when combined with RT and a surgical intent to preserve a critical structure (such as vessels, major nerves, or bone), margins of less than 1 cm may still be adequate. As covered in the article by Dr Delaney elsewhere in this issue, wide excision and RT result in acceptable LR rates and good limb functionality in most patients.

PATHOLOGIC ASSESSMENT OF THE STS RESECTION MARGIN

The pathologic assessment of the resected STS specimen is not only important for the diagnosis (histologic type and grade), which affects prognosis but also the margin status, which determines the need for additional therapy (eg, reresection, RT). Therefore, it is recommended that all STS specimens be evaluated by a pathology team with expertise in this disease. There are also some inherent difficulties and limitations to margin assessment and pathologic evaluation of STS specimens. Ex vivo, the relationship of the tumor to surrounding structures can change greatly. Surrounding muscle fibers do not remain isometric after being transected. This muscular retraction and opening of intermuscular planes can lead to margins being inaccurately defined as close or positive. Therefore, communication between the surgeon and the pathologist who will be grossing the tumor is imperative. Ideally, the surgeon should take the resection specimen to pathology and anatomically orient it for the pathologist. The specimen should be fresh, not formalin fixed, to allow the pathologist to examine/measure the specimen undistorted, take photographs, and perform specialized cytogenetic and molecular diagnostic studies, if indicated. The resection specimen should be measured in 3 dimensions and the closest distance for each margin from the edge of the tumor should be noted. The surgeon should also identify any margins of concern, the anticipated closest margin, and other structures critical to the pathologic assessment, such as margins that contain intact fascia. Margin inking should be performed only after photographs of the specimen are obtained and a thorough gross examination has been performed. Permanent blocks should be taken to definitely include the closest gross resection margin and the deep margin, when appropriate.[11] It is recommended that even wide gross margins (>3 cm) from the tumor be assessed for some histologic subtypes known to infiltrate significant distances (myxofibrosarcoma and epithelioid sarcoma).

In certain circumstances, intraoperative frozen section assessment is informative and helps guide therapy. It may help define clinically suspicious tissues when resecting recurrent or previously irradiated tumors. If there is an intraoperative positive margin, consideration could be given to resection of additional tissue or perhaps intraoperative radiation. However, frozen section analysis can often be time consuming, technically challenging, and inaccurate (eg, atypical spindle cells in an irradiated prior surgical site). Therefore, unless the results of the frozen section will change the intraoperative management, it is not routinely recommended for STS resections.

MARGIN STATUS AND LR

Given the rarity and heterogeneity of STS combined with the inconsistent use of adjuvant therapies, accurate data on LR rates are difficult to obtain and interpret. **Table 1** summarizes the results of several large STS series. LR rates vary greatly from 7% to 42%. Currently, the expected risk for LR in the modern multimodality STS treatment era should be less than or equal to 20%.

Most of the STS literature shows that a positive resection margin is associated with an increased risk for LR (**Table 2**). Biologically, this makes sense, but what is more intriguing is the natural history of a positive-margin resection. Most positive margins do not lead to an LR. In a Memorial Sloan Kettering Cancer Center (MSKCC) analysis of 2084 patients with STS (all anatomic sites), 22% (n = 460) had a positive resection margin.[1] The LR rate for a positive margin was 28%. Conversely, that means that 72% of positive-margin resections did not result in an LR. Although the LR rate was significantly higher for positive versus negative-margin resections (risk ratio [RR] 2.4), 15% of negative margins still had an LR. In a similar large series from MD Anderson Cancer Center (MDACC) of 1091 patients with STS, 22.6% of patients (n = 247) had a positive resection margin despite all gross tumor being clinically resected.[18] However, only 15.9% of all 1091 patients (n = 173) developed an LR. Consequently, although a positive resection margin places a patient with STS at a higher risk for LR, it is still more likely that an LR will not occur.

It has also been observed that not all positive margins are the same. Gerrand and colleagues[25] classified positive margins after combined limb salvage STS surgery and radiotherapy into 4 distinct categories to quantify the risk for LR: (1) a positive margin for a low-grade, well-differentiated liposarcoma; (2) a planned positive margin at an anatomically critical structure (bone, vessel, or nerve) preserved at the time of surgery; (3) a positive margin after reexcision for a prior unplanned excision at an outside center; (4) an unplanned positive margin (surgical error). Positive margins in the first 2 categories were associated with low rates of LR (4.2% and 3.6%, respectively), whereas the third and fourth categories had a higher risk for LR (31.6% and 37.5%, respectively).

What about the distance of the negative resection margin? Are all negative margins equal? In an analysis by Novais and colleagues[24] of 248 patients with STS, margins

Table 1
LR rates for published soft tissue sarcoma series

Series	Time Frame	Patients (n)	Follow-Up (y)	High Grade (%)	Deep (%)	Radiation (%)	Amputation (%)	LR (%)
Stotter et al,[6] 1990	1982–1987	175	3	60	77	55	0	42
Pisters et al,[12] 1996	1982–1994	1041	4	65	76	40	10	17
Coindre et al,[13] 1996	1980–1989	546	5	84	79	56	4	29
Yang et al,[14] 1998	1983–1991	132	10	70	NR	50	0	11
Baldini et al,[15] 1999	1970–1994	74	10.5	49	66	0	0	7
Karakousis and Driscoll,[16] 1999	1977–1994	194	3	86	88	42	7	15
Trovik et al,[9] 2001	1986–1995	1331	6	78	66	24	10	17
Zagars et al,[17] 2003	1960–1999	1225	9.5	71	N/A	>95	0	41
Lahat et al,[18] 2008	1997–2007	1091	4.4	67	64	44	N/A	16

Abbreviations: LR, local recurrence; N/A, not available; NR, not reported; y, years.

Table 2
The relationship of margin status to LR and survival for published soft tissue sarcoma series

Series	Time Frame	Patients (n)	Margin Classification	LR	Survival
Tanabe et al[19]	1970–1987	95	Positive vs negative	Microscopic positive surgical margin or intraoperative tumor violation had increased LR	Neither positive margin nor LR adversely affected survival
Lewis et al[20]	1982–1994	495	Positive vs negative	On univariate and multivariate analysis, LR was associated with positive microscopic margins (RR 2.1)	On multivariate analysis, a positive microscopic margin had a worse metastasis-free survival
Pisters et al[12]	1982–1994	1041	Positive (within 1 mm) vs negative	Positive margin was an independent prognostic factor for LR (RR 1.8)	On multivariate analysis, positive margin was an adverse factor for DSS
Lewis et al[21]	1982–1995	911	Positive vs negative	On univariate and multivariate, a positive microscopic margin was associated with increased LR	Positive microscopic margin was associated with distant recurrence and decreased DSS
Zagars et al[17]	1960–1999	1225	Positive, negative, or uncertain	On univariate and multivariate analysis, margin status was a major factor contributing to local control (RR 2.5)	Positive margin was associated with decreased disease-free survival
Stojadinovic et al[1]	1982–2000	2084	Positive vs negative	Positive margin nearly doubled the risk of LR	Positive margin increased the risk of disease-related death
Dickinson et al[22]	1987–2002	279	Contaminated, >20 mm, 10–19 mm, 5–9 mm, 1–4 mm, <1 mm	Contaminated margins had higher rates of LR	Failure to obtain an uncontaminated margin was associated with decreased OS
Liu et al[23]	1997–2007	181	0–1 mm, 1–4 mm, 5–9 mm, 10–19 mm, 20–29 mm, ≥30 mm	Margin<10 mm was an independent risk factor for LR	Margin<10 mm was associated with decreased metastasis-free and DSS
Novais et al[24]	1995–2008	248	Positive at ink, ≤2 mm, >2 mm but ≤2 cm, >2 cm	Margin≤2 mm was associated with increased LR	Inadequate surgical margin (≤2 mm) was associated with decreased OS

Abbreviations: DSS, disease-specific survival; LR, local recurrence; OS, overall survival; RR, risk ratio.

were categorized as positive at ink, less than or equal to 2 mm, greater than 2 mm but less than or equal to 2 cm, or greater than 2 cm. Margins less than or equal to 2 mm had a higher risk for LR compared with margins greater than 2 cm (12% vs <2.4%, P = .002) Baldini and colleagues[15] found that the 10-year local control rate for the closest margin being less than 1 cm was lower than for a margin greater than or equal to 1 cm (87% vs 100%, respectively, P = .04). Dickinson and colleagues[22] also showed a relationship between the extent of the negative resection margin and LR (**Fig. 1**).

POSITIVE MARGINS, LR, AND SURVIVAL

Since the shift away from amputation to multimodality limb salvage, the relationship between positive margins, LR, and survival has been an area of controversy. Intuitively, LR should not be a major causative factor for distant metastases; otherwise, amputation should cure most patients with STS.[26] Historically, this was not the case. However, as noted earlier, positive margins are associated with an increased risk for LR. In addition, many STS series have shown a strong relationship between LR and decreased survival.[18,21,24,27,28] Therefore, if positive margins increase the risk for LR and LR is associated with decreased survival, then the key question becomes, by the transitive property, does a positive-margin resection directly increase the chance of dying from an STS? Alternatively, is a positive-margin resection simply a marker of a more aggressive tumor biology, which, in itself, has a higher risk for metastases?

In a study by Lewis and colleagues[20] of patients with localized primary STS, a positive-margin resection was associated with a decreased disease-specific survival (DSS) on univariate analysis. On multivariate analysis, positive margins still affected 5-year DSS (RR 4.6, P = .02) and metastasis-free survival (P = .009). In the previously noted large MSKCC series, margin positivity was associated with a decreased 5-year DSS (70% vs 80% for positive vs negative, respectively; $P<.001$).[1] Similarly, the large MDACC series showed that the 5-year disease-specific mortality was significantly lower for negative versus positive-margin resections (18% vs 31%, $P<.0001$, **Fig. 2**), but this effect was limited to high-grade tumors.[18] In a different retrospective MDACC review of 1225 patients with localized STS treated with conservative surgery and radiation, resection margins were defined as positive if tumor was present at the inked resection margin, negative if tumor was not present at the margin (regardless of the distance of the negative margin), and uncertain if the report did not comment explicitly on the margin.[17] A negative resection margin was associated with a better DFS on multivariate regression analysis compared with positive/uncertain margins. The

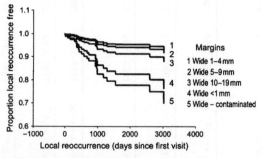

Fig. 1. LR-free survival based on soft tissue sarcoma resection margin status. (*From* Dickinson IC, Whitwell DJ, Battistuta D, et al. Surgical margin and its influence on survival in soft tissue sarcoma. ANZ J Surg 2006;76(3):107; with permission.)

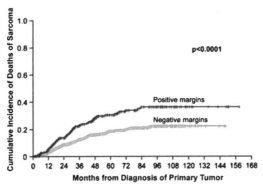

Fig. 2. Cumulative incidence of sarcoma-related deaths by postresection margin status as a function of time from initial diagnosis. (*From* Lahat G, Tuvin D, Wei C, et al. New perspectives for staging and prognosis in soft tissue sarcoma. Annals of Surgical Oncology 2008;15(10):2745; with permission.)

impact of margin status on survival for several STS series is also summarized in **Table 2**.

Which data would support the notion that positive margins and even LR have no direct impact on STS survival? In the MDACC series mentioned earlier, on multivariable analysis, margin status was no longer a significant variable for DSS if the presence/absence of LR was included.[18] In the MSKCC series, 23% of the 2084 patients with STS developed a distant recurrence, but most (75%) had negative resection margins.[1] In the study by Dickinson and colleagues,[22] the patients who underwent a radical resection (typically very advanced tumors) had a worse prognosis, suggesting that the tumor biology was more important than the resection margins (**Fig. 3**).[22] Other indirect evidence includes the beneficial effects of adjuvant RT on LR, but not OS. Two studies of adjuvant brachytherapy radiation showed a lower risk for LR compared with surgery alone, but no difference in OS.[12,29] Yang and colleagues[14] found that external beam RT significantly decreased the probability of LR, but it did not improve OS.

An additional question is whether an extremity STS LR can directly lead to mortality. An Italian series of 997 consecutive patients with extremity STS analyzed outcome

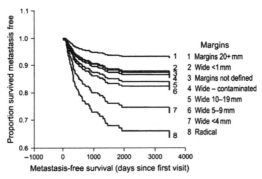

Fig. 3. Metastasis-free survival based on soft tissue sarcoma resection margin status. (*From* Dickinson IC, Whitwell DJ, Battistuta D, et al. Surgical margin and its influence on survival in soft tissue sarcoma. ANZ J Surg 2006;76(3):107; with permission.)

based on resection margin status.[30] An R0 resection was performed in 87.7% compared with 11.7% R1 resections (tumor <1 mm from the resection margin). RT was performed in 44.6% and chemotherapy in 19.9% The 5-year and 10-year LR rates were 10% and 12%, respectively, for R0 resection versus 26% and 30%, respectively, for R1 resection ($P<.001$). The 5-year and 10-year disease-specific mortalities were also significantly different at 16% and 19%, respectively, for R0 resection versus 29% and 38%, respectively, for R1 resection ($P = .0003$). In the R0 group, all deaths were caused by distant metastases. However, in the R1 group, 17% of deaths were secondary to locoregional recurrence, primarily proximally. On Cox proportional hazard modeling, margin status was significantly associated with both DSS ($P = .002$) and LR-free survival ($P = .001$), but not distant metastasis-free survival ($P = .979$). The investigators concluded that surgical margin status directly affected survival primarily through LR at proximal sites.

One of the better analyses of the relationships between STS surgical margins, LR, and outcome is by Trovik and colleagues.[9] A review of the Scandinavian Sarcoma Group Register identified 559 adult patients with extremity and truncal STS treated with surgery alone (no radiation or chemotherapy). Surgical resection margins were categorized as inadequate or adequate, extrapolating from the Enneking system. As with most other studies, the risk for LR was associated with margin status (RR 2.9, $P<.001$). A Cox regression analysis for time to metastasis and risk factors for metastases was performed using 2 models: model A with variables identified on univariate analysis (LR not included), and model B, which also included LR as a time-dependent variable. In model A, surgical margin status was not statistically significant, suggesting that it was not a surrogate for LR. In model B, LR was significant (RR 4.4, $P<.001$), but margin status was not significant (RR 1.1, $P = .6$). In subgroup analyses of high risk (both high grade and size >7 cm) or low risk (none or only 1 of these features), LR was again a significant risk factor in both groups, but margin status was not significant. The investigators concluded that "…an inadequate surgical margin is a risk factor for local recurrence but not for metastasis. High malignancy grade and large tumor size, but not surgical margins, are together with local recurrence important and independent prognostic factors for metastasis. The well-known association between local recurrence and metastasis must be interpreted as non-causal; highly malignant tumors combine both local and distant aggressiveness."[9]

MANAGEMENT OF THE POSITIVE RESECTION MARGIN

Although a positive resection margin may not directly influence OS, there is a clear association with the risk for LR. As with any primary solid tumor, local control of the primary tumor is the first step to potential cure. Therefore, the goal of surgical resection for a primary STS should be to obtain a negative-margin resection within the confines of preserving reasonable functionality and quality of life. In practice, there a two categories of a positive margin resection. The first is an anticipated positive margin that was intentional to preserve a critical structure (vessels, nerve, or bone). In this situation, additional surgery, including amputation, is not indicated because the most appropriate oncologic procedure has already been performed. Instead, strong consideration should be given to the addition of RT to further reduce the risk for LR. The other category of positive-margin resection is following an unplanned non-oncologic excision (so-called whoops procedure) or a planned oncologic procedure in which the final resection margins were positive but additional tissue could still be resected with acceptable morbidity. In this case, the most appropriate approach is to consider repeat resection in an attempt to obtain negative margins.

In a study by Lin and colleagues,[31] 115 patients with hand and foot STS who had inadequate or unplanned excisions were analyzed based on whether or not they underwent a subsequent definitive wide excision versus no additional surgery. The 10-year LR-free survival for the patients who underwent a definitive reexcision was significantly better (88%) compared with the patients who did not receive additional surgery (53%, $P = .05$, **Fig. 4**). In a series of 666 patients with STS who presented to MDACC after prior complete macroscopic tumor resection at an outside institution, 44% (n = 295) underwent reresection versus 56% (n = 371) who had no further surgery.[32] All patients received adjuvant RT. The margin status for the patients who did not undergo reresection was 32% negative, 13% positive, and 56% unknown. Final resection margin status for the patients undergoing reresection was 87% negative, 12% positive, and 1% unknown. For the patients having reresection who previously had positive margins, 35% had residual tumor on final pathology (20% gross disease). Even 33% (4/12) of patients who had negative margins on the original excision had residual tumor on reresection. The 5-year, 10-year, and 15-year local control rates for reresection were 85%, 85%, and 82%, respectively, versus 78%, 73%, and 73%, respectively, for patients who did not undergo reresection ($P = .03$). On multivariate regression analysis, reresection status was significantly associated with decreased LR (RR 1.6, $P = .041$).

Perhaps the most provocative study in support of a definitive surgical reexcision following an unplanned STS resection is by Lewis and colleagues.[33] In this retrospective review of 1092 patients, 685 patients were referred directly to MSKCC and underwent a single definitive surgical resection (1 operation) compared with 407 patients who underwent a reresection at MSKCC after undergoing a prior unplanned excision without wide margins at another institution (2 operations). Demographically, the single-operation group had a significantly higher rate of high-grade and deep tumors. The rate of final positive resection margins was also significantly higher in the single-operation versus 2-operation group (25.5% vs 9.1%, respectively, $P = .01$). Although there was no difference in LR-free survival between the 2 groups ($P = .7$), the 2-operation group had a significantly higher 5-year metastasis-free survival compared with the single-definitive-operation group (83% vs 63%, respectively, $P = .0001$). The

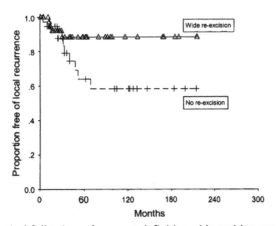

Fig. 4. LR-free survival following subsequent definitive wide excision versus no additional surgery for patients undergoing an unplanned excision of a hand or foot sarcoma. (*From* Lin PP, Guzel VB, Pisters PW, et al. Surgical management of soft tissue sarcomas of the hand and foot. Cancer 2002;95(4):855; with permission.)

survival difference was most significant in the high-risk patients who were American Joint Commission on Cancer (AJCC) stage III (>5 cm, deep, high grade) (P = .005). The investigators admitted that they did not have an explanation for these results. Potential theories included an unidentified referral or selection bias, that reresection resulted in a more complete removal of clinically occult residual tumor (although there was no difference in LR), or perhaps an immunostimulatory effect by the second surgery. Regardless, the findings of this study support the recommendation that patients who have undergone an unplanned excision of their STS should be strongly considered for a definitive surgical reresection in an attempt to obtain negative margins.

Although limb-sparing surgery is the standard of care for extremity STS, approximately 5% of patients require amputation because the gross tumor cannot be adequately resected with preservation of limb function.[34,35] However, given the rarity of STS and the long-term functional implications of amputation, all patients being considered for this procedure should be assessed at a sarcoma center with multidisciplinary expertise in the treatment of this disease.

SUMMARY

A negative-margin surgical resection is the potentially curative treatment of an STS. The data clearly show that a positive-margin resection is associated with an increased risk for LR. An LR can be morbid for the patient, not only functionally but also psychologically. For extremity STS, LR may even lead to amputation.

Positive-margin STS resections are generally divided into 2 categories. The first is a positive margin following an unplanned excision in which no attempt was made to perform an oncologic resection with widely negative margins. This situation is under the control of the surgeon. Surgical reresection to obtain negative margins not only reduces the risk for LR, but there is also some evidence to suggest that survival may be better. In this scenario, it is not appropriate to simply use adjuvant RT to replace inadequate, nononcologic surgery.

In contrast, even at centers with significant sarcoma expertise, approximately 20% to 25% of oncologic STS resections have positive margins on final pathology. This is not because of bad surgery. Rather, a conscious decision is often made to accept a very close or microscopically positive margin near a critical vascular, neurologic, or bony structure as a trade-off to preserve limb functionality and quality of life. Consequently, any attempt at reresection to obtain negative margins would likely be morbid, possibly even requiring amputation. Therefore, accepting the positive margin with a known increased risk for LR and also considering the role of radiation to reduce that risk is the most appropriate therapy.

Although a positive-margin resection is associated with a higher chance of LR and LR has been associated with a decreased DSS, there are no conclusive scientific data that accepting a positive-margin resection in the setting of a well-planned multimodality limb salvage treatment approach jeopardizes the patient's chance of cure. First, most positive-margin resections do not recur. Second, most of the LRs in large sarcoma series are in patients who had a negative-margin resection. Third, for extremity STS, there are no data showing that OS was better in the amputation era compared with the modern multimodality limb salvage era.

In conclusion, physicians treating STS have 2 equally important, but apparently separate, clinical challenges: obtaining local control of the primary tumor and curing the patient. But the disconnect between these 2 issues is no more apparent than in the LR-free survival and OS data for extremity STS based on AJCC stage. The 5-year local recurrence-free survival for stage I, II, and III is 88%, 82%, and 83%, respectively.[36] Despite significant differences in risk factors for LR (size, grade, and depth) between these groups, local control is good and similar across all 3 stages. In contrast, the 5-year OS for stage I, II, and III is very different at 90%, 81%, and 56%, respectively. It is difficult to imagine that LR is driving most distant metastases, especially in the high-risk stage III patients in whom local control is significantly better than OS. Rather, it is more logical to assume that the features that make a biologically aggressive STS at high risk for metastasizing hematogenously may also increase the chance for having a positive-margin resection and an LR. Therefore, the relationship between margin status, LR, and survival seems to be correlation as opposed to causation.

ACKNOWLEDGMENTS

We would like to thank Richard Cheney, MD, Chair - Department of Pathology at Roswell Park Cancer Institute, for contributing his knowledge on pathologic assessment of the sarcoma specimen.

REFERENCES

1. Stojadinovic A, Leung DH, Hoos A, et al. Analysis of the prognostic significance of microscopic margins in 2,084 localized primary adult soft tissue sarcomas. Ann Surg 2002;235(3):424.
2. Rosenberg SA, Tepper J, Glatstein E, et al. The treatment of soft-tissue sarcomas of the extremities: prospective randomized evaluations of (1) limb-sparing surgery plus radiation therapy compared with amputation and (2) the role of adjuvant chemotherapy. Ann Surg 1982;196(3):305.
3. Limb-Sparing Treatment of Adult Soft-Tissue Sarcomas and Osteosarcomas. NIH Consensus Statement Online 1984;5(6):1–7.
4. Enneking WF, Spanier SS, Goodman MA. A system for the surgical staging of musculoskeletal sarcoma. Clin Orthop Relat Res 1980;(153):106.
5. Mc Kee MD, Liu DF, Brooks JJ, et al. The prognostic significance of margin width for extremity and trunk sarcoma. J Surg Oncol 2004;85(2):68–76.
6. Stotter AT, A'hern R, Fisher C, et al. The influence of local recurrence of extremity soft tissue sarcoma on metastasis and survival. Cancer 1990;65(5):1119–29.
7. Emrich LJ, Ruka W, Driscoll DL, et al. The effect of local recurrence on survival time in adult high-grade soft tissue sarcomas. J Clin Epidemiol 1989;42(2):105–10.
8. Rydholm A, Rooser B. Surgical margins for soft-tissue sarcoma. J Bone Joint Surg Am 1987;69(7):1074–8.
9. Trovik C, Bauer H, Alvegård T, et al. Surgical margins, local recurrence and metastasis in soft tissue sarcomas: 559 surgically-treated patients from the Scandinavian Sarcoma Group Register. Eur J Cancer 2000;36(6):710–6.
10. NCCN clinical practice guidelines in oncology. Soft tissue sarcoma. Version 1.2011. National Comprehensive Cancer Network, Inc; 2011.
11. Fisher C, Montgomery EA, Thway K. Biopsy interpretation of soft tissue tumors. Philadelphia: Wolters Kluwer Health/Lippincott Williams & Wilkins; 2011.
12. Pisters P, Harrison LB, Leung D, et al. Long-term results of a prospective randomized trial of adjuvant brachytherapy in soft tissue sarcoma. J Clin Oncol 1996; 14(3):859.
13. Coindre JM, Terrier P, Bui NB, et al. Prognostic factors in adult patients with locally controlled soft tissue sarcoma. A study of 546 patients from the French Federation of Cancer Centers Sarcoma Group. J Clin Oncol 1996;14(3):869–77.

14. Yang JC, Chang AE, Baker AR, et al. Randomized prospective study of the benefit of adjuvant radiation therapy in the treatment of soft tissue sarcomas of the extremity. J Clin Oncol 1998;16(1):197.
15. Baldini EH, Goldberg J, Jenner C, et al. Long-term outcomes after function-sparing surgery without radiotherapy for soft tissue sarcoma of the extremities and trunk. J Clin Oncol 1999;17(10):3252.
16. Karakousis CP, Driscoll DL. Treatment and local control of primary extremity soft tissue sarcomas. J Surg Oncol 1999;71:155–61.
17. Zagars GK, Ballo MT, Pisters PW, et al. Prognostic factors for patients with localized soft-tissue sarcoma treated with conservation surgery and radiation therapy. Cancer 2003;97(10):2530–43.
18. Lahat G, Tuvin D, Wei C, et al. New perspectives for staging and prognosis in soft tissue sarcoma. Ann Surg Oncol 2008;15(10):2739–48.
19. Tanabe KK, Pollock RE, Ellis LM, et al. Influence of surgical margins on outcome in patients with preoperatively irradiated extremity soft tissue sarcomas. Cancer 1994;73(6):1652–9.
20. Lewis JJ, Leung D, Casper ES, et al. Multifactorial analysis of long-term follow-up (more than 5 years) of primary extremity sarcoma. Arch Surg 1999;134(2):190.
21. Lewis JJ, Leung D, Heslin M, et al. Association of local recurrence with subsequent survival in extremity soft tissue sarcoma. J Clin Oncol 1997;15(2):646.
22. Dickinson IC, Whitwell DJ, Battistuta D, et al. Surgical margin and its influence on survival in soft tissue sarcoma. ANZ J Surg 2006;76(3):104–9.
23. Liu CY, Yen CC, Chen WM, et al. Soft tissue sarcoma of extremities: the prognostic significance of adequate surgical margins in primary operation and reoperation after recurrence. Ann Surg Oncol 2010;17(8):2102–11.
24. Novais EN, Demiralp B, Alderete J, et al. Do surgical margin and local recurrence influence survival in soft tissue sarcomas? Clin Orthop Relat Res 2010;468(11):3003–11.
25. Gerrand C, Wunder J, Kandel R, et al. Classification of positive margins after resection of soft-tissue sarcoma of the limb predicts the risk of local recurrence. J Bone Joint Surg Br 2001;83(8):1149.
26. Brennan MF. Local recurrence in soft tissue sarcoma: more about the tumor, less about the surgeon. Ann Surg Oncol 2007;14(5):1528–9.
27. Sabolch A, Feng M, Griffith K, et al. Risk factors for local recurrence and metastasis in soft tissue sarcomas of the extremity. Am J Clin Oncol 2011 [Epub ahead of print].
28. Eilber FC, Rosen G, Nelson SD, et al. High-grade extremity soft tissue sarcomas: factors predictive of local recurrence and its effect on morbidity and mortality. Ann Surg 2003;237(2):218.
29. Brennan MF, Hilaris B, Shiu MH, et al. Local recurrence in adult soft-tissue sarcoma: a randomized trial of brachytherapy. Arch Surg 1987;122(11):1289.
30. Gronchi A, Lo Vullo S, Colombo C, et al. Extremity soft tissue sarcoma in a series of patients treated at a single institution: local control directly impacts survival. Ann Surg 2010;251:506–11.
31. Lin PP, Guzel VB, Pisters PW, et al. Surgical management of soft tissue sarcomas of the hand and foot. Cancer 2002;95(4):852–61.
32. Zagars GK, Ballo MT, Pisters PW, et al. Surgical margins and reresection in the management of patients with soft tissue sarcoma using conservative surgery and radiation therapy. Cancer 2003;97:2544–53.
33. Lewis JJ, Leung D, Espat J, et al. Effect of reresection in extremity soft tissue sarcoma. Ann Surg 2000;231(5):655.

34. Clark MA, Thomas JM. Amputation for soft-tissue sarcoma. Lancet Oncol 2003; 4(6):335–42.
35. Ghert MA, Abudu A, Driver N, et al. The indications for and the prognostic significance of amputation as the primary surgical procedure for localized soft tissue sarcoma of the extremity. Ann Surg Oncol 2005;12(1):10–7.
36. Edge SB, Byrd DR, Compton CC, et al. Soft tissue sarcoma. In: Edge SB, Byrd DR, Compton CC, et al, editors. AJCC Cancer staging manual. 7th edition. New York: Springer; 2010. p. 291–6.

Pulmonary Metastasectomy for Soft Tissue Sarcoma

Richard Smith, MD[a,b], Todd L. Demmy, MD[c,d],*

KEYWORDS

- Soft tissue sarcoma • Pulmonary metastases
- Metastasectomy • Sarcomatous metastases
- Pulmonary resection

The American Cancer Society predicts 10,520 new cases and 3920 deaths from soft tissue sarcoma (STS) for 2010.[1] STS disseminates primarily via the hematogenous route, although lymphatic spread does occur with certain subtypes.[2] The lung is the most common metastatic site in most large series, accounting for up to 80% of metastases.[3] The rate of metastatic disease primarily depends on tumor grade and ranges from 10% for low grade to 30% for intermediate and greater than 50% for high grade.[4] Approximately 70% of pulmonary metastases occur within the first 2 years after primary tumor resection.[5]

The median overall survival (OS) for pulmonary metastatic disease with current multidisciplinary treatment is approximately 12 to 14 months.[6–9] Pulmonary metastasectomy (PM) represents the only potentially curative treatment for patients with STS and lung metastases.[10,11] The first PM was described by Weinlechner[12] in 1882 when 2 lesions were removed incidentally during resection of a chest wall sarcoma. Alexander and Haight[13] were the first to show a survival benefit and describe criteria for resection, which include control of the primary tumor, absence of extrathoracic disease, and sufficient pulmonary reserve. These criteria remain valid to this day.

PM is the accepted standard therapy for a small subset of patients with STS with resectable disease and favorable tumor biology. This standard is based on an

The authors have nothing to disclose.
[a] Department of Surgery, Tripler Army Medical Center, 1 Jarrett White Road, Honolulu, HI 96859, USA
[b] Department of Surgery, Cancer Research Center of Hawaii, 1236 Lauhala Street, Honolulu, HI 96813, USA
[c] Department of Thoracic Surgery, Roswell Park Cancer Institute, Elm & Carlton Streets, Buffalo, NY 14263, USA
[d] Department of Surgery, State University of New York-Buffalo, 100 High Street, Buffalo, NY 14203, USA
* Corresponding author. Department of Thoracic Surgery, Roswell Park Cancer Institute, Elm & Carlton Streets, Buffalo, NY 14263.
E-mail address: Todd.Demmy@roswellpark.org

Surg Oncol Clin N Am 21 (2012) 269–286
doi:10.1016/j.soc.2011.12.001
1055-3207/12/$ – see front matter

abundance of retrospective studies showing improved survival with complete resection versus historical controls without resection. Despite aggressive surgical management, recurrence rates are still greater than 50%.[14]

IMAGING EVALUATION

Ideally, chest imaging identifies all metastatic lesions and is able to differentiate benign from malignant processes. However, inflammatory conditions can often mimic metastases.[15] Pulmonary metastases are usually described as multiple round nodules of varying size with indistinct borders, spiculation, pleural thickening, and inhomogeneity of the surrounding lung parenchyma.[16] Certain sarcomas commonly present with calcified metastases (osteogenic/chondrogenic and synovial sarcoma) and can be mistaken for benign processes such as granulomatous disease.[17]

Chest radiography remains an important modality for the staging and surveillance of patients with STS. The low cost, universal availability, and excellent safety record are the reasons for its continued utility. Despite being very specific for the identification of pulmonary metastases, sensitivity is limited.[18]

Computed Tomographic Scan

The improved sensitivity of computed tomographic (CT) scans over plain chest radiography has framed a more recent debate regarding the best screening modality for pulmonary metastases. The advent of standard CT imaging followed by helical CT with thin sectioning has increased the detection rate (sensitivity) for small pulmonary nodules.[19] Sliding thin-slab maximum intensity projection (MIP) techniques create 2-dimensional representations of the initial thin sections to differentiate pulmonary vessels from nodules (by showing the whole course of the vessel within the slice), thus decreasing false-positives.[20,21] The addition of computer-aided diagnosis (CAD) also increases sensitivity of pulmonary nodule detection as compared with standard CT scanning.[22]

Although the addition of MIP or CAD to multidetector CT has shown an increased sensitivity for nodule detection, few studies have demonstrated a positive impact of these aids in the setting of pathologically proved malignancy. Of the few studies available, all but one deal with lung cancer.[23–25] The lone study of both MIP and CAD in patients undergoing PM showed increased sensitivity per patient and per nodule.[25] This increased sensitivity was valid only for nodules that are 5 mm or smaller. Colorectal, renal, and hepatocellular cancers comprised two-thirds of the patients, so this study may not be applicable to patients with STS.

CT scanning demonstrates pulmonary nodules in 33% of newly diagnosed patients with STS, and approximately 80% of these turn out to be metastases.[26] Indeterminate lesions 10 mm or smaller make up 21% of nodules, of which 28% are metastatic.[19] Patients having only lesions smaller than 5 mm that remain stable over 6 months enjoy similar survival as those with normal CT scan results.[19,26,27] Magnetic resonance imaging has a sensitivity similar to that of conventional CT scan, so offers no specific advantage.[17]

Positron Emission Tomography

Molecular imaging using positron emission tomography (PET) with fludeoxyglucose F 18 (^{18}F FDG-PET) is a useful modality for the differentiation of benign from malignant soft tissue masses. Moreover, it is also a useful tool to evaluate response to therapy.[28] [18]F FDG-PET uptake can also predict prognosis and grade of the primary tumor.[29,30] However, the sensitivity of ^{18}F FDG-PET for STS pulmonary metastases is relatively low (50%–86.5%) than that of CT (95.1%–100%).[31–34] Specificity is similar for both modalities.[31–34] Because of the lack of spatial resolution of ^{18}F FDG-PET, its fusion with CT into an integrated PET/CT improves sensitivity and specificity beyond what either achieves alone in malignancies such as lung cancer. Iagaru and colleagues[32] examined 106 patients with osseous sarcoma and STS who underwent dedicated chest CT. Seventy-six of these patients underwent a dedicated PET, and the remaining 30 patients had hardware-fused PET/CT imaging. There was no difference in sensitivity or specificity between the 2 groups, concluding that PET/CT does not add power to diagnostic value over PET alone. Although PET/CT imaging may have improved since this study, PET/CT for STS is challenged by the lack of intravenous contrast and single breath-hold technique for the CT portion of the technology. Furthermore, lower-grade sarcomas do not have reliably high glucose metabolism (standardized uptake value) like malignancies for which PET/CT has proved superior.

FACTORS AFFECTING PATIENT SELECTION FOR PM

PM represents the only potentially curative treatment for patients with STS and lung metastases. Despite aggressive surgical management, recurrence rates remain greater than 50%. Therefore, careful consideration is necessary when determining whether or not a patient will benefit from surgical intervention. Appropriate patient selection requires that the following criteria be confirmed, within reason. First, the primary tumor is controlled or controllable. Second, extrathoracic disease is absent. Third, there is sufficient pulmonary reserve to tolerate complete resection of all disease. Last, complete resection is achievable.

Synchronous Pulmonary Metastases

The proportion of patients with STS who initially present with synchronous pulmonary metastases is approximately 10%.[4,35–38] There are only 2 studies specifically addressing patients with STS and synchronous disease.[39] Kane and colleagues[39] reviewed 48 patients with synchronous metastatic disease, of which 30 had pulmonary metastases. Thirteen of these patients underwent PM, and there was no significant difference in median survival between patients who underwent resection and who did not. Ferguson and colleagues[38] studied 112 patients who presented with synchronous metastases. Eighty-eight (79%) patients had pulmonary metastases, 18 of whom underwent PM. Median OS was 9 months for all patients presenting with synchronous pulmonary metastases. There were 3 long-term survivors from the 18 patients who underwent resection, but this did not show significance on multivariate analysis. A similar study by Liebl and colleagues[40] did not specifically look at synchronous presentation but included it in a univariate analysis. Patients with synchronous disease had a median survival of 21 months versus 40 months with metachronous metastases. The poor outcome for synchronous metastases could be predicted, considering the known negative impact of short disease-free interval (DFI) in STS PM series.[6,41–43] Given the poor results of PM in these cases, patients with synchronous metastatic disease should instead be considered for clinical trials or initial chemotherapy to assess response and tumor biology.[11,38,39]

Impact of Primary Tumor Local Recurrence on PM

Limited data exist regarding the impact of prior local recurrence (LR) on outcome after subsequent PM. In Pisters and colleagues'[44] large series of patients with STS, the overall rate of distant metastatic disease was 22%. About 30% of these patients developed metastases synchronously with or after an LR. However, LR did not significantly affect postmetastasis survival. In Billingsley and colleagues'[9] study, 18% of patients with metastasis had an LR as a preceding event and another 6% had metastases synchronous with an LR. In contrast to Pisters and colleagues' cohort, patients with an LR were twice as likely to die from their metastases. Chen and colleagues[45] examined their experience with PM in 23 patients with STS who underwent complete resection. Multivariate analysis showed that 10 patients who had a prior LR were 20 times more likely to die than patients without a prior recurrence.[45] Ueda and colleagues[46] also found a better 5-year OS in patients without an associated LR (30.0% for LR vs 12.5% for no recurrence). This was significant on univariate analysis but was not subjected to multivariate analysis. Although these are only small series on which to base decisions, the presence of an LR may diminish the anticipated therapeutic benefit of PM.

Extrathoracic Metastatic Disease

Studies on patients with a combination of pulmonary and extrathoracic metastases are also limited. In a large series of extremity STS with distant metastases, nonlung metastases had a postresection survival similar to pulmonary metastases.[9] In Blackmon and colleagues'[47] study, 36.2% of patients undergoing PM had prior synchronous or metachronous extrathoracic metastases. The most common sites of extrathoracic metastases were spine, bone, soft tissue, liver, abdomen, brain, and pelvis. Three groups were compared: pulmonary metastases only, pulmonary metastases plus synchronous or prior extrathoracic metastases, and pulmonary metastases plus subsequent metachronous extrathoracic metastases. There was no difference in survival between the group with resected pulmonary tumor only and that with resected pulmonary plus synchronously or previously resected extrathoracic tumor. Survival was very poor in patients undergoing PM in whom the extrathoracic metastases could not be completely resected. This finding supports resection of pulmonary metastases and extrathoracic metastases only when the tumor can be completely resected. In this situation, one could expect survival similar to isolated pulmonary metastases.

Adequate Pulmonary Reserve

In general, PM is associated with low morbidity and mortality rates. Patients with STS lung metastases do not typically have chronic obstructive pulmonary disease or other cardiopulmonary comorbidities common in patients with lung cancer. In addition, the PM surgical procedures are generally conservative wedge resections, and most lesions are peripherally located. Wedge resections or segmentectomies are performed in 73% to 86% of cases.[5,42,43,46,48,49] Perioperative mortality is typically 0.0% to 3.7%.[5,41–43,46,48,49] Perioperative morbidity ranges from 6% to 14%.[42,46,50,51]

Completeness of Surgical Resection

Consistently, the factor most significantly associated with improved survival after PM is complete resection of the metastatic disease.[6,41,43,52] In Smith and colleagues'[43] study, the median OS for R0 (complete) resection was 22 months, 11.5 months for R1 (microscopically positive margin) resection, and 9.5 months for R2 (grossly positive margin) resection. In Billingsley and colleagues'[6] study, the median survival after complete resection was 33 months versus 16 months for an incomplete resection.

SURGICAL APPROACH TO PM

Planning a PM for STS requires careful consideration of each case individually. Rather than relying on 1 approach, it is probably most advantageous to have all techniques available to fit to each unique situation. The ideal approach depends on the surgeon's experience and the anatomic locations of the metastases. In addition, minimally invasive surgical options are being used with increasing frequency, representing a potentially curative and repeatable procedure with less pain, decreased hospital stay, and faster recovery.

Median Sternotomy

The main advantage of median sternotomy is simultaneous access to both pleural cavities. Another advantage over standard posterolateral thoracotomy is less pain and respiratory compromise. However, the heart limits exposure of the hila and left lower lobe. The more posterior segments are also less accessible.[53,54] Although infrequent, sternal wound complications cause high morbidity.[53]

Transsternal Thoracotomy

Bilateral anterolateral thoracotomies with transsternal extension (clamshell incision) offer optimal exposure, especially the hila and left lower lobe, as compared with median sternotomy.[53,54] Although postoperative pain is greater than with median sternotomy, because of the sternal release, less force is applied to fewer rib interspaces and may lead to less pain than bilateral traditional thoracotomies.[53,54] This approach does sacrifice the bilateral internal thoracic arteries and precludes their use for flap reconstruction or revascularization procedures.

Posterolateral Thoracotomy

A traditional posterolateral thoracotomy through the fifth or sixth interspace provides excellent exposure for unilateral and hilar lesions. There was initially some controversy surrounding performing unilateral thoracotomy for patients with unilateral disease by imaging. The National Cancer Institute reported a higher yield of occult pulmonary nodules for median sternotomy than unilateral thoracotomy. Despite finding more disease, survival was not improved.[55] Younes and colleagues[56] compared patients who underwent bilateral thoracotomies for bilateral disease with patients initially noted to have unilateral disease undergoing unilateral thoracotomy in whom the condition recurred in the contralateral lung. The investigators found that delaying contralateral thoracotomy until disease became radiologically apparent did not affect OS.

Video-Assisted Thoracoscopic Surgery

Experience with minimally invasive thoracic surgical approaches continues to grow as the techniques and supporting technology mature. Video-assisted thoracoscopic surgery (VATS) offers patients with STS and lung metastases a potentially curative and repeatable treatment option with low perioperative morbidity. The rationale for VATS comes from several factors identified in PM series. The initial concerns regarding VATS centered on the lack of manual palpation of the lungs like what is performed during open thoracotomy. Additional nonimaged but palpable nodules were identified in 42% of patients undergoing PM.[57] In a recent series using multidetector CT scan with thin cuts and fused PET/CT, 37% of patients had missed nodules found with manual palpation; 18% had a missed malignant nodule.[58] This view that VATS was an inferior approach because of missed metastases was further supported by results of a prospective trial of VATS followed by confirmatory thoracotomy showing that additional malignant lesions were identified in 56% of patients at confirmatory thoracotomy.[59]

A contrary view of VATS arose from the knowledge that a significant neoplastic burden remains in micronodules (1–2 mm) that are beyond the detection of both CT and manual palpation. Consequently, the intrathoracic recurrence rate in open thoracotomy series has been as high as 50% to 69%.[49,60,61] Even in a median sternotomy series in which both thoracic cavities were palpated, the intrathoracic recurrence rate was nearly 40%.[62] Roth and colleagues[55] also showed that occult contralateral disease existed in 40% of patients with STS undergoing PM via sternotomy as compared with unilateral thoracotomy, but the choice of unilateral exploration did not affect survival.

In series comparing VATS with thoracotomy, both modalities showed similar survival.[63–65] Carballo and colleagues[64] examined 171 patients with various malignancies (47% sarcoma). Of those, 135 underwent thoracotomy and 36 underwent VATS. The 5-year OS was 58.8% in the thoracotomy group and 69.6% in the VATS group (**Fig. 1**). The subgroup with the highest survival included patients with sarcoma undergoing VATS. Gossot and colleagues[65] examined STS PM with characteristics favorable for VATS: 2 or less lesions per lung field, maximum tumor dimension of 3 cm, wedge resection technically possible, and no extraparenchymal disease. A total of 31 patients underwent a VATS procedure and were compared with 29 patients with similar tumor characteristics who underwent standard thoracotomy. There was no difference in OS, disease-free survival (DFS), or ipsilateral recurrence rates. Mutsaerts and colleagues[66] compared patients with a solitary nodule identified on preoperative CT prospectively undergoing VATS with similar historical controls who had undergone confirmatory thoracotomy. There was no difference in DFS or OS between the 2 groups at 2 years.

Potential benefits of VATS over standard thoracotomy include reduced postoperative morbidity, pain, decreased hospital stay, and earlier return to work.[65–69] Another important potential benefit of VATS for STS PM is based on the role of repeat metastasectomy in some patients. In Weiser and colleagues'[51] study, 35% of their patients with STS undergoing an initial PM underwent a second thoracic exploration for recurrence and 37% of that subgroup underwent a third thoracic exploration. Kondo and

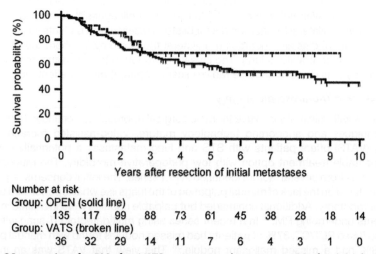

Number at risk
Group: OPEN (solid line)
    135   117   99   88   73   61   45   38   28   18   14
Group: VATS (broken line)
    36   32   29   14   11   7   6   4   3   1   0

Fig. 1. OS comparison for PM after VATS versus open thoracotomy. OS after initial metastasectomy for the 2 procedure groups. Median OS was 47.3 months. The actuarial OS rates for VATS and open thoracotomy, respectively, are the following: 1-year OS at 91.7% and 87.4%; 3-year OS at 69.6% at 67.9%; and 5-year OS at 69.6% and 58.8%. (*From* Carballo M, Maish MS, Jaroszewski DE, et al. Video-assisted thoracic surgery (VATS) as a safe alternative for the resection of pulmonary metastases: a retrospective cohort study. J Cardiothorac Surg 2009;4:13; with permission.)

colleagues[70] specifically observed the benefit of VATS in repeat PM. Patients were placed into 4 groups: group A (previous VATS/present VATS), group B (previous VATS/present thoracotomy), group C (previous thoracotomy/present VATS), and group D (previous thoracotomy/present thoracotomy). Operative times, bleeding, and chest tube drainage in group D were significantly longer than those for the other 3 groups.

Size, depth, and consistency of the metastasis influence the ability to identify the nodule thoracoscopically. A variety of methods have been used to aid in the intraoperative identification of nodules, including intraoperative ultrasonography; percutaneous injection of dye, contrast material, or radionuclides; percutaneous hook wire; wire coil placement; and transbronchial localization.[71–76] Preoperative localization is most helpful in the following situations: maximum diameter of nodule of 5 mm or less, maximum diameter to minimum distance between visceral pleura and inferior border of the nodule of 0.5 or less, low-density or ground-glass appearance of the lesion, and location in anatomically difficult areas such as basilar segments of the lower lobes.[77] The most common method involves the use of the hook wire or suture system. This technique is highly successful with a low complication rate and has the added benefit over other techniques of offering a means of retraction intraoperatively.[77,78]

Emerging technologies such as navigational bronchoscopy have been used to localize lung nodules for stereotactic radiosurgery, so it is conceivable that this technology could be used to aid in surgical excision also in the future.[71]

EXTENT OF RESECTION

The goal of PM is a negative margin with preservation of lung parenchyma. Given the peripheral nature of STS metastases, this can often be accomplished with wedge resection. However, multiple lesions within a lobe or centrally located lesions may require more extensive resections.

Pneumonectomy

The International Registry of Lung Metastases reported on 5206 patients undergoing PM.[79] Pneumonectomy was performed in 4% (171 patients). With pneumonectomy, there was a 4% preoperative mortality and a 5-year OS of 20% for patients who underwent complete resection (as compared with no survivors beyond 25 months in the group that underwent incomplete resection). The pneumonectomy group was dominated by patients with STS who had a 5-year OS of 30% if they underwent complete resection. Long-term survival is possible with pneumonectomy in carefully selected patients when the expected outcome is balanced against the increased morbidity and mortality rates.

Extended Resection

Patients with STS requiring concurrent en bloc chest wall, pericardial, or diaphragm resection have a significantly shorter median OS than those undergoing only subpleural resection.[42,43,46] However, when subjected to multivariant analysis, this difference loses significance, likely secondary to an association with incomplete resection.[42,43] Therefore, extended resection with en bloc structures may be potentially curative if negative margins can be achieved.

Thoracic Lymph Node Dissection

The role of thoracic lymph node dissection in PM has been studied in mixed populations of patients with epithelial cancer, sarcomatous cancer, germ cell cancer, renal cancer, and melanoma undergoing pulmonary resection. The 5-year OS with lymph node involvement is 0% to 14%, compared with 36% to 60% with no lymph node involvement.[49,80,81] Pfannschmidt and colleagues[82] reported on 245 patients who underwent PM along with systematic hilar and mediastinal lymph node dissection. Of these patients, 69 had osteogenic or STS pulmonary metastases. The prevalence of lymph node involvement for patients with sarcoma was 23%. The median survival for the sarcoma group was 47 months for node-negative, 18.3 months for N1, and 22 months for N2 involvement ($P = .036$). Hilar and mediastinal lymph node involvement is a poor prognostic indicator and, if identified preoperatively, should be considered a relative contraindication to resection. In the case of occult metastases, further studies of systematic nodal dissection to determine the true prevalence should be considered.

RECURRENCE AND REPEATED PM

The intrathoracic recurrence rate after a complete resection PM for any malignancy is 42% to 70%.[41,45,49,60] Even if only patients undergoing median sternotomy are considered, the recurrence rate is still approximately 40%, despite exploring both pleural cavities.[55,62] The 5-year OS following repeated resection is typically 36% to 57%.[49,51,83,84] This compares favorably with patients undergoing their first PM procedure. Although most of these series include all types of cancers, these conclusions are probably also valid for patients with STS because similar results are seen in smaller sarcoma-specific series (**Table 1**).

Long-term survival is possible with repeated PM and is appropriate when a complete resection can be achieved. In fact, for patients with STS undergoing PM, repeated metastasectomy has been associated with improved survival.[5,40,43,85] To be able to undergo repeated metastasectomy likely identifies a subset of patients with STS with a good physiologic condition and favorable tumor biology.

There is no upper limit to the number of PM resections a patient can undergo. Jaklitsch and colleagues[84] found that 5-year OS remained greater than 33% for up to 4 procedures. With 5 or more procedures, the ability to maintain control of the

Table 1
Results of repeat sarcoma PM

Author	Year	Patients	Median Survival Incomplete Resection (mo)	Median Survival Complete Resection (mo)	Significant Factors
Casson et al[100]	1991	39	7	28	Resectability, number of metastases
Pogrebniak et al[50]	1991	43	10	25	R0, DFI, age
Rizzoni et al[101]	1986	29	7	20	Resectability, TDT, DFI, number of metastases
Weiser et al[51]	2000	86	6	51	R0, number of metastases, size largest metastasis, grade

Abbreviations: DFI, disease-free interval between first and second pulmonary resection; R0, complete resection; TDT, tumor doubling time.

intrathoracic metastases became very low and median survival dropped to 8 months. The investigators' conclusion was that repeating procedures are indicated as long as removal of all clinically apparent disease is practical.[84]

LONG-TERM SURVIVAL FOLLOWING PM

To date, no randomized prospective trials have been performed showing superior survival for STS PM as compared with best medical/supportive care. However, several published studies have shown a 5-year actuarial OS of 23% to 43% in patients who have undergone complete resection.[5,6,41,42,45,46,48,49] These studies are summarized in **Table 2**. Even accounting for selection bias for being a candidate for PM, these outcomes still significantly exceed what can be accomplished with traditional systemic chemotherapy.

Complete resection is the most important predictor of survival after PM with a median survival of 19 to 33 months for patients who underwent complete resection as compared with 6 to 16 months for incomplete resection.[6,42,43,49,52,60,85] The next most common but less consistent factors are DFI and the number of metastases. van Geel and colleagues[86] examined both DFI and the number of metastases in a meta-analysis using a crude method of combination of P values and found that DFI was a significant predictor of postresection survival but the number of metastases was not. The studies included in the meta-analysis used varying definitions for DFI, making the exact cutoff difficult to define. However, a DFI of 7 months or less was clearly a bad prognostic factor.[86] Other studies have shown that the number of metastases does affect postmetastasectomy survival.[42,48,49,87–89] However, there is no number above which resection is prohibitive. Pastorino and colleagues[49] showed that even with 10 or more metastases, 5-year survival was still 26%. Functionally, the number of metastases is likely closely associated with determining a patient's "resectability." Other factors identified on multivariate analyses that negatively affect survival are increasing age; male sex; histologic findings of malignant fibrous histiocytoma, liposarcoma, and malignant peripheral nerve tumor; high-grade primary tumor; decreased doubling time; diameter of the largest metastasis; LR; and truncal primary tumor site.[6,41,42,45,52,85,87,89,90] None of these additional factors have been consistent across all studies.

ADJUVANT THERAPY AFTER PM
Radiation Therapy

Routine adjuvant thoracic radiation has no defined role in the management of patients with STS with completely resected pulmonary metastases.[91] In available PM series, radiation therapy (external beam as well as brachytherapy techniques) has occasionally been used after a positive margin resection or for residual gross disease.[43,60] In Smith and colleagues'[43] study, radiation therapy was used in patients with positive margins or cases involving associated extrapleural resections. Median survival was 16 months for patients receiving radiation therapy versus 26 months when radiation was not used ($P = .98$).

Chemotherapy

For patients with STS and metastatic disease, the 2 most commonly used chemotherapy agents are doxorubicin and ifosfamide. Both have response rates around 25%, with a median OS of about 12 months.[92] In a study combining 7 trials from the European Organization for Research and Treatment of Cancer, including patients with metastatic and locally advanced nonresectable STS, the chemotherapy response

Table 2
Survival results for STS PM series

Author	Year	Number of Patients	Percentage of Survival[a] (%)	Predictive Factors and Comments[b]
Roth et al[89]	1985	67	—	Number of nodules on tomogram, DFI, tumor doubling time
Jablons et al[52]	1989	63	26.8	DFI, sex, resectability, trunk location for primary
Lanza et al[93]	1991	24	22	—
Casson et al[42]	1992	68	25.8	≥4 nodules on CT, malignant fibrous histiocytoma histology
Verazin et al[85]	1992	61	21[a]	LR, resectability, number of thoracotomies, DFI ([a]actual 5-year survival)
Gadd et al[60]	1993	135	38[a]	([a]2-year OS)
Mentzer et al[88]	1993	77	26	Number of metastases, resection vs chemotherapy (univariate analysis)
Saltzman et al[90]	1993	49	39	Size of largest nodule, series includes osteogenic and STS metastases
Ueda et al[46]	1993	23	24.8	Synovial histology, grade, extrapleural invasion (univariate analysis)
Choong et al[87]	1995	214	40	Size of largest metastasis, ≥2 metastases, DFI
van Geel et al[41]	1996	255	38	DFI, grade, R0, age
Pastorino[49]	1997	1917	31	DFI, number of metastases
Billingsley et al[6]	1999	161	37	Resectability, DFI, grade, age, liposarcoma and malignant peripheral nerve tumor histologies
Rehders et al[5]	2007	61	25	von Recklinghausen disease or other preexisting condition (univariate analysis)
Chen et al[45]	2009	23	43	Repeated metastasectomy, LR
Garcia Franco et al[48]	2009	20	23.1	DFI, ≥4 nodules resected, Ewing sarcoma histology (univariate analysis)
Smith et al[43]	2009	74	18[a]	DFI, R0 ([a]actual 5-year survival)

Abbreviation: R0, complete resection.

[a] Actuarial 5-year OS following complete resection except as noted in comments section.

[b] Multivariate analysis except as noted in comments section.

rate was 21%, with a complete clinical response rate of 5%.[8] Consolidation chemotherapy in the setting of pulmonary metastases should be considered primarily palliative, although a small subset achieves long-term survival.[8,88] Blay and colleagues[8] showed a 5-year survival of 8% in patients with metastatic and locally advanced non-resectable STS.

When given as a neoadjuvant for patients who are potential candidates for PM, chemotherapy response rate of 30% to 50% with complete clinical responses of 12% to 21% have been reported.[88,93] Lanza and colleagues[93] examined 24 patients undergoing neoadjuvant chemotherapy followed by PM. A complete radiographic response was seen in 21%, 29% had a partial response, and 50% had no change or disease progression. In all the complete responders the condition subsequently recurred, and they underwent PM. There was no difference in postmetastasectomy survival between patients who had a complete response, a partial response, and progressive disease. A retrospective study examining prognostic factors in 214 patients with STS undergoing PM found that systemic chemotherapy was a negative predictor for survival on univariate analysis.[87] This difference disappeared on multivariate analysis, suggesting a potential selection bias for the patients receiving chemotherapy. Canter and colleagues[94] reported on 136 patients undergoing PM for their first lung metastasis. Perioperative chemotherapy was given to 51 patients as compared with surgery alone in 85 patients. Median postmetastasectomy disease-specific survival was 24 months for the perioperative chemotherapy group versus 33 months for the surgery-alone group ($P = .19$). The lack of a survival benefit from chemotherapy is consistent across all STS pulmonary metastases series in which it was included in the analysis.[5,40,43,46,52,60,85,87] Without a randomized trial, the true impact of perioperative chemotherapy in patients with STS undergoing PM is unanswered. However, the available evidence suggests minimal, if any, benefit over surgical resection alone.

NONSURGICAL ABLATIVE THERAPY FOR PULMONARY METASTASES

Radiofrequency ablation (RFA) has become an accepted, relatively safe, and effective treatment modality for a subset of suboptimal surgical candidates with pulmonary or hepatic metastatic colorectal cancer as well as for unresectable non–small cell lung cancer.[95] Reports on RFA for STS lung metastases are limited to a few patients usually included as part of larger studies observing multiple malignancies. Nakamura and colleagues[96] examined 20 patients with pulmonary metastases from musculoskeletal sarcomas undergoing RFA. Complete ablation was achieved in 55% of patients. The 1- and 3-year survival rates were 88.9% and 59.2%, respectively, in the group that underwent complete ablation versus 29.6% and 0%, respectively, in the group that underwent incomplete ablation ($P<.02$). The 3-year survival in the group that underwent complete ablation was similar to reported survivals for PM. However, because of a high recurrence rate (particularly with lesions >3 cm), RFA for lung metastases should only be used in select patients who are unable to undergo surgical PM.[97]

In contrast to traditional external beam radiation, the development of stereotactic body radiotherapy (SBRT) has increased enthusiasm for radioablation of pulmonary metastases. SBRT uses external surrogate markers (fiducial) or image guidance in the treatment room for localization of the tumor and delivers a single or small number (hypofractionated) of large radiation doses. A high dose can be used safely because the treated volumes are small with tight margins, and the technique uses multiple small dose beams that collectively deliver the large dose to the target.[98] At these high doses, the radiation becomes tissue ablative. Dhakal and colleagues[99] treated patients with

STS pulmonary metastasis who were nonsurgical candidates using SBRT and noted a 3-year local control rate of 82%. Median OS for patients undergoing SBRT was 2.1 years, which was much higher than the 0.6 years for patients not treated with SBRT. SBRT seems to provide good local control that could potentially translate into prolonged survival. However, given the wide variety of treatment techniques and dose fraction variations in the literature, there is no consensus for a standard approach using SBRT for pulmonary metastases.[98]

SUMMARY

Although there are no randomized prospective trials showing the absolute benefit for PM in patients with STS, 5-year survivals of up to 40% in patients who have undergone complete resection as compared with less than 10% in patients not undergoing resection offer fairly compelling evidence. The available studies also clearly show that incomplete resections are rarely beneficial. Therefore, the single most important consideration when evaluating potential patients with PM is the likelihood of achieving a complete resection. DFI, the next most commonly identified prognostic factor, serves as a surrogate for tumor biology and should also be considered in the decision-making process. This prognostic factor is most ominous when equal to 0, that is, synchronous disease. A reasonable approach to patients presenting with synchronous disease or early multiple pulmonary nodules is to consider a limited course of neoadjuvant chemotherapy to determine the pace of disease progression before considering resection.[5,47] The number of metastases is also a frequently identified prognostic factor, but there is no absolute limit to the maximum number of resected metastases because long-term survival is possible even with more than 10 metastases.[49] Long-term survival often requires multiple repeated PMs, given the high recurrence rate. This underscores the importance of pulmonary parenchymal preservation for future procedures. The long-term outcomes of VATS seem the same as for traditional open approaches, and repeating VATS procedures can be less complicated. Also, novel minimally invasive techniques, such as RFA or SBRT, can be considered when pulmonary reserve or medical comorbidities preclude PM.

REFERENCES

1. Jemal A, Siegel R, Xu J, et al. Cancer statistics, 2010. CA Cancer J Clin 2010; 60(5):277–300.
2. Weiss S, Goldblum J, editors. Enzinger and Weiss's soft tissue tumors. 5th edition. Philadelphia: Mosby Elsevier; 2008.
3. Potter DA, Glenn J, Kinsella T, et al. Patterns of recurrence in patients with high-grade soft-tissue sarcomas. J Clin Oncol 1985;3(3):353–66.
4. Coindre JM, Terrier P, Guillou L, et al. Predictive value of grade for metastasis development in the main histologic types of adult soft tissue sarcomas: a study of 1240 patients from the French Federation of Cancer Centers Sarcoma Group. Cancer 2001;91(10):1914–26.
5. Rehders A, Hosch SB, Scheunemann P, et al. Benefit of surgical treatment of lung metastasis in soft tissue sarcoma. Arch Surg 2007;142(1):70–5 [discission: 76].
6. Billingsley KG, Burt ME, Jara E, et al. Pulmonary metastases from soft tissue sarcoma: analysis of patterns of diseases and postmetastasis survival. Ann Surg 1999;229(5):602–10 [discussion: 610–2].
7. Italiano A, Mathoulin-Pelissier S, Cesne AL, et al. Trends in survival for patients with metastatic soft-tissue sarcoma. Cancer 2011;117(5):1049–54.

8. Blay JY, van Glabbeke M, Verweij J, et al. Advanced soft-tissue sarcoma: a disease that is potentially curable for a subset of patients treated with chemotherapy. Eur J Cancer 2003;39(1):64–9.
9. Billingsley KG, Lewis JJ, Leung DH, et al. Multifactorial analysis of the survival of patients with distant metastasis arising from primary extremity sarcoma. Cancer 1999;85(2):389–95.
10. Temple LK, Brennan MF. The role of pulmonary metastasectomy in soft tissue sarcoma. Semin Thorac Cardiovasc Surg 2002;14(1):35–44.
11. King JJ, Fayssoux RS, Lackman RD, et al. Early outcomes of soft tissue sarcomas presenting with metastases and treated with chemotherapy. Am J Clin Oncol 2009;32(3):308–13.
12. Weinlechner J. Tumoren an der brustwand und deren behnadlung resection der rippeneroffnung der brusthohle und partielle entfernung der lunge. Weiner Med Wrsch 1882;32:589–91 [in German].
13. Alexander J, Haight C. Pulmonary resection for solitary metastatic sarcomas and carcinomas. Surg Gynecol Obstet 1947;85(2):129–46.
14. Sonett JR. Pulmonary metastases: biologic and historical justification for VATS. Video assisted thoracic surgery. Eur J Cardiothorac Surg 1999;16(Suppl 1): S13–5 [discussion: S15–6].
15. Seemann MD, Seemann O, Luboldt W, et al. Differentiation of malignant from benign solitary pulmonary lesions using chest radiography, spiral CT and HRCT. Lung Cancer 2000;29(2):105–24.
16. Seo JB, Im JG, Goo JM, et al. Atypical pulmonary metastases: spectrum of radiologic findings. Radiographics 2001;21(2):403–17.
17. Maile CW, Rodan BA, Godwin JD, et al. Calcification in pulmonary metastases. Br J Radiol 1982;55(650):108–13.
18. Christie-Large M, James SL, Tiessen L, et al. Imaging strategy for detecting lung metastases at presentation in patients with soft tissue sarcomas. Eur J Cancer 2008;44(13):1841–5.
19. Rissing S, Rougraff BT, Davis K. Indeterminate pulmonary nodules in patients with sarcoma affect survival. Clin Orthop Relat Res 2007;459:118–21.
20. Ginsberg MS, Panicek DM. Subcentimeter pulmonary nodules detected in patients with sarcoma. Sarcoma 2000;4(1–2):63–6.
21. Gruden JF, Ouanounou S, Tigges S, et al. Incremental benefit of maximum-intensity-projection images on observer detection of small pulmonary nodules revealed by multidetector CT. AJR Am J Roentgenol 2002;179(1):149–57.
22. Rubin GD, Lyo JK, Paik DS, et al. Pulmonary nodules on multi-detector row CT scans: performance comparison of radiologists and computer-aided detection. Radiology 2005;234(1):274–83.
23. Goo JM, Kim HY, Lee JW, et al. Is the computer-aided detection scheme for lung nodule also useful in detecting lung cancer? J Comput Assist Tomogr 2008; 32(4):570–5.
24. Armato SG 3rd, Li F, Giger ML, et al. Lung cancer: performance of automated lung nodule detection applied to cancers missed in a CT screening program. Radiology 2002;225(3):685–92.
25. Park EA, Goo JM, Lee JW, et al. Efficacy of computer-aided detection system and thin-slab maximum intensity projection technique in the detection of pulmonary nodules in patients with resected metastases. Invest Radiol 2009;44(2): 105–13.
26. Nakamura T, Matsumine A, Niimi R, et al. Management of small pulmonary nodules in patients with sarcoma. Clin Exp Metastasis 2009;26(7):713–8.

27. Robertson PL, Boldt DW, De Campo JF. Paediatric pulmonary nodules: a comparison of computed tomography, thoracotomy findings and histology. Clin Radiol 1988;39(6):607–10.
28. Bastiaannet E, Groen H, Jager PL, et al. The value of FDG-PET in the detection, grading and response to therapy of soft tissue and bone sarcomas; a systematic review and meta-analysis. Cancer Treat Rev 2004;30(1):83–101.
29. Eary JF, Conrad EU, Bruckner JD, et al. Quantitative [F-18]fluorodeoxyglucose positron emission tomography in pretreatment and grading of sarcoma. Clin Cancer Res 1998;4(5):1215–20.
30. Schwarzbach MH, Dimitrakopoulou-Strauss A, Willeke F, et al. Clinical value of [18-F] fluorodeoxyglucose positron emission tomography imaging in soft tissue sarcomas. Ann Surg 2000;231(3):380–6.
31. Lucas JD, O'Doherty MJ, Wong JC, et al. Evaluation of fluorodeoxyglucose positron emission tomography in the management of soft-tissue sarcomas. J Bone Joint Surg Br 1998;80(3):441–7.
32. Iagaru A, Chawla S, Menendez L, et al. 18F-FDG PET and PET/CT for detection of pulmonary metastases from musculoskeletal sarcomas. Nucl Med Commun 2006;27(10):795–802.
33. Gerth HU, Juergens KU, Dirksen U, et al. Significant benefit of multimodal imaging: PET/CT compared with PET alone in staging and follow-up of patients with Ewing tumors. J Nucl Med 2007;48(12):1932–9.
34. Franzius C, Daldrup-Link HE, Sciuk J, et al. FDG-PET for detection of pulmonary metastases from malignant primary bone tumors: comparison with spiral CT. Ann Oncol 2001;12(4):479–86.
35. Bauer HC, Trovik CS, Alvegard TA, et al. Monitoring referral and treatment in soft tissue sarcoma: study based on 1,851 patients from the Scandinavian Sarcoma Group Register. Acta Orthop Scand 2001;72(2):150–9.
36. Nijhuis PH, Schaapveld M, Otter R, et al. Epidemiological aspects of soft tissue sarcomas (STS)—consequences for the design of clinical STS trials. Eur J Cancer 1999;35(12):1705–10.
37. Komdeur R, Hoekstra HJ, van den Berg E, et al. Metastasis in soft tissue sarcomas: prognostic criteria and treatment perspectives. Cancer Metastasis Rev 2002;21(2):167–83.
38. Ferguson PC, Deheshi BM, Chung P, et al. Soft tissue sarcoma presenting with metastatic disease: outcome with primary surgical resection. Cancer 2011; 117(2):372–9.
39. Kane JM, Finley JW, Driscoll D, et al. The treatment and outcome of patients with soft tissue sarcomas and synchronous metastases. Sarcoma 2002;6(2): 69–73.
40. Liebl LS, Elson F, Quaas A, et al. Value of repeat resection for survival in pulmonary metastases from soft tissue sarcoma. Anticancer Res 2007;27(4C): 2897–902.
41. van Geel AN, Pastorino U, Jauch KW, et al. Surgical treatment of lung metastases: the European Organization for Research and Treatment of Cancer-Soft Tissue and Bone Sarcoma Group study of 255 patients. Cancer 1996;77(4): 675–82.
42. Casson AG, Putnam JB, Natarajan G, et al. Five-year survival after pulmonary metastasectomy for adult soft tissue sarcoma. Cancer 1992;69(3):662–8.
43. Smith R, Pak Y, Kraybill W, et al. Factors associated with actual long-term survival following soft tissue sarcoma pulmonary metastasectomy. Eur J Surg Oncol 2009;35(4):356–61.

44. Pisters PW, Leung DH, Woodruff J, et al. Analysis of prognostic factors in 1,041 patients with localized soft tissue sarcomas of the extremities. J Clin Oncol 1996;14(5):1679–89.
45. Chen F, Fujinaga T, Sato K, et al. Significance of tumor recurrence before pulmonary metastasis in pulmonary metastasectomy for soft tissue sarcoma. Eur J Surg Oncol 2009;35(6):660–5.
46. Ueda T, Uchida A, Kodama K, et al. Aggressive pulmonary metastasectomy for soft tissue sarcomas. Cancer 1993;72(6):1919–25.
47. Blackmon SH, Shah N, Roth JA, et al. Resection of pulmonary and extrapulmonary sarcomatous metastases is associated with long-term survival. Ann Thorac Surg 2009;88(3):877–84 [discussion: 884–5].
48. Garcia Franco CE, Algarra SM, Ezcurra AT, et al. Long-term results after resection for soft tissue sarcoma pulmonary metastases. Interact Cardiovasc Thorac Surg 2009;9(2):223–6.
49. Long-term results of lung metastasectomy: prognostic analyses based on 5206 cases. The International Registry of Lung Metastases. J Thorac Cardiovasc Surg 1997;113(1):37–49.
50. Pogrebniak HW, Roth JA, Steinberg SM, et al. Reoperative pulmonary resection in patients with metastatic soft tissue sarcoma. Ann Thorac Surg 1991;52(2):197–203.
51. Weiser MR, Downey RJ, Leung DH, et al. Repeat resection of pulmonary metastases in patients with soft-tissue sarcoma. J Am Coll Surg 2000;191(2):184–90 [discussion: 190–1].
52. Jablons D, Steinberg SM, Roth J, et al. Metastasectomy for soft tissue sarcoma. Further evidence for efficacy and prognostic indicators. J Thorac Cardiovasc Surg 1989;97(5):695–705.
53. Demmy TL, Dunn KB. Surgical and nonsurgical therapy for lung metastasis: indications and outcomes. Surg Oncol Clin N Am 2007;16(3):579–605, ix.
54. Kaifi JT, Gusani NJ, Deshaies I, et al. Indications and approach to surgical resection of lung metastases. J Surg Oncol 2010;102(2):187–95.
55. Roth JA, Pass HI, Wesley MN, et al. Comparison of median sternotomy and thoracotomy for resection of pulmonary metastases in patients with adult soft-tissue sarcomas. Ann Thorac Surg 1986;42(2):134–8.
56. Younes RN, Gross JL, Deheinzelin D. Surgical resection of unilateral lung metastases: is bilateral thoracotomy necessary? World J Surg 2002;26(9):1112–6.
57. McCormack PM, Ginsberg KB, Bains MS, et al. Accuracy of lung imaging in metastases with implications for the role of thoracoscopy. Ann Thorac Surg 1993;56(4):863–5 [discussion: 865–6].
58. Cerfolio RJ, McCarty T, Bryant AS. Non-imaged pulmonary nodules discovered during thoracotomy for metastasectomy by lung palpation. Eur J Cardiothorac Surg 2009;35(5):786–91 [discussion: 791].
59. McCormack PM, Bains MS, Begg CB, et al. Role of video-assisted thoracic surgery in the treatment of pulmonary metastases: results of a prospective trial. Ann Thorac Surg 1996;62(1):213–6 [discussion: 216–7].
60. Gadd MA, Casper ES, Woodruff JM, et al. Development and treatment of pulmonary metastases in adult patients with extremity soft tissue sarcoma. Ann Surg 1993;218(6):705–12.
61. Mountain CF, McMurtrey MJ, Hermes KE. Surgery for pulmonary metastasis: a 20-year experience. Ann Thorac Surg 1984;38(4):323–30.
62. Pastorino U, Valente M, Gasparini M, et al. Median sternotomy and multiple lung resections for metastatic sarcomas. Eur J Cardiothorac Surg 1990;4(9):477–81.

63. Nakajima J, Takamoto S, Tanaka M, et al. Thoracoscopic surgery and conventional open thoracotomy in metastatic lung cancer. Surg Endosc 2001;15(8): 849–53.

64. Carballo M, Maish MS, Jaroszewski DE, et al. Video-assisted thoracic surgery (VATS) as a safe alternative for the resection of pulmonary metastases: a retrospective cohort study. J Cardiothorac Surg 2009;4:13.

65. Gossot D, Radu C, Girard P, et al. Resection of pulmonary metastases from sarcoma: can some patients benefit from a less invasive approach? Ann Thorac Surg 2009;87(1):238–43.

66. Mutsaerts EL, Zoetmulder FA, Meijer S, et al. Long term survival of thoracoscopic metastasectomy vs metastasectomy by thoracotomy in patients with a solitary pulmonary lesion. Eur J Surg Oncol 2002;28(8):864–8.

67. Landreneau RJ, Wiechmann RJ, Hazelrigg SR, et al. Effect of minimally invasive thoracic surgical approaches on acute and chronic postoperative pain. Chest Surg Clin N Am 1998;8(4):891–906.

68. Hazelrigg SR, Nunchuck SK, Landreneau RJ, et al. Cost analysis for thoracoscopy: thoracoscopic wedge resection. Ann Thorac Surg 1993;56(3):633–5.

69. Tschernko EM, Hofer S, Bieglmayer C, et al. Early postoperative stress: videoassisted wedge resection/lobectomy vs conventional axillary thoracotomy. Chest 1996;109(6):1636–42.

70. Kondo R, Hamanaka K, Kawakami S, et al. Benefits of video-assisted thoracic surgery for repeated pulmonary metastasectomy. Gen Thorac Cardiovasc Surg 2010;58(10):516–23.

71. Harley DP, Krimsky WS, Sarkar S, et al. Fiducial marker placement using endobronchial ultrasound and navigational bronchoscopy for stereotactic radiosurgery: an alternative strategy. Ann Thorac Surg 2010;89(2):368–73 [discussion: 373–4].

72. Powell TI, Jangra D, Clifton JC, et al. Peripheral lung nodules: fluoroscopically guided video-assisted thoracoscopic resection after computed tomographyguided localization using platinum microcoils. Ann Surg 2004;240(3):481–8 [discussion: 488–9].

73. Moon SW, Wang YP, Jo KH, et al. Fluoroscopy-aided thoracoscopic resection of pulmonary nodule localized with contrast media. Ann Thorac Surg 1999;68(5): 1815–20.

74. Nomori H, Horio H, Naruke T, et al. Fluoroscopy-assisted thoracoscopic resection of lung nodules marked with lipiodol. Ann Thorac Surg 2002;74(1):170–3.

75. Mattioli S, D'Ovidio F, Daddi N, et al. Transthoracic endosonography for the intraoperative localization of lung nodules. Ann Thorac Surg 2005;79(2):443–9 [discussion: 443–9].

76. Shinagawa N, Yamazaki K, Onodera Y, et al. CT-guided transbronchial biopsy using an ultrathin bronchoscope with virtual bronchoscopic navigation. Chest 2004;125(3):1138–43.

77. Nakashima S, Watanabe A, Obama T, et al. Need for preoperative computed tomography-guided localization in video-assisted thoracoscopic surgery pulmonary resections of metastatic pulmonary nodules. Ann Thorac Surg 2010;89(1):212–8.

78. Dendo S, Kanazawa S, Ando A, et al. Preoperative localization of small pulmonary lesions with a short hook wire and suture system: experience with 168 procedures. Radiology 2002;225(2):511–8.

79. Koong HN, Pastorino U, Ginsberg RJ. Is there a role for pneumonectomy in pulmonary metastases? International Registry of Lung Metastases. Ann Thorac Surg 1999;68(6):2039–43.

80. Veronesi G, Petrella F, Leo F, et al. Prognostic role of lymph node involvement in lung metastasectomy. J Thorac Cardiovasc Surg 2007;133(4):967–72.
81. Loehe F, Kobinger S, Hatz RA, et al. Value of systematic mediastinal lymph node dissection during pulmonary metastasectomy. Ann Thorac Surg 2001;72(1): 225–9.
82. Pfannschmidt J, Klode J, Muley T, et al. Nodal involvement at the time of pulmonary metastasectomy: experiences in 245 patients. Ann Thorac Surg 2006; 81(2):448–54.
83. Kandioler D, Kromer E, Tuchler H, et al. Long-term results after repeated surgical removal of pulmonary metastases. Ann Thorac Surg 1998;65(4):909–12.
84. Jaklitsch MT, Mery CM, Lukanich JM, et al. Sequential thoracic metastasectomy prolongs survival by re-establishing local control within the chest. J Thorac Cardiovasc Surg 2001;121(4):657–67.
85. Verazin GT, Warneke JA, Driscoll DL, et al. Resection of lung metastases from soft-tissue sarcomas. A multivariate analysis. Arch Surg 1992;127(12):1407–11.
86. van Geel AN, Rm van Der Sijp J, Schmitz PI. Which soft tissue sarcoma patients with lung metastases should not undergo pulmonary resection? Sarcoma 2002; 6(2):57–60.
87. Choong PF, Pritchard DJ, Rock MG, et al. Survival after pulmonary metastasectomy in soft tissue sarcoma. Prognostic factors in 214 patients. Acta Orthop Scand 1995;66(6):561–8.
88. Mentzer SJ, Antman KH, Attinger C, et al. Selected benefits of thoracotomy and chemotherapy for sarcoma metastatic to the lung. J Surg Oncol 1993;53(1): 54–9.
89. Roth JA, Putnam JB Jr, Wesley MN, et al. Differing determinants of prognosis following resection of pulmonary metastases from osteogenic and soft tissue sarcoma patients. Cancer 1985;55(6):1361–6.
90. Saltzman DA, Snyder CL, Ferrell KL, et al. Aggressive metastasectomy for pulmonic sarcomatous metastases: a follow-up study. Am J Surg 1993;166(5): 543–7.
91. Abdalla EK, Pisters PW. Metastasectomy for limited metastases from soft tissue sarcoma. Curr Treat Options Oncol 2002;3(6):497–505.
92. Sleijfer S, Seynaeve C, Verweij J. Using single-agent therapy in adult patients with advanced soft tissue sarcoma can still be considered standard care. Oncologist 2005;10(10):833–41.
93. Lanza LA, Putnam JB Jr, Benjamin RS, et al. Response to chemotherapy does not predict survival after resection of sarcomatous pulmonary metastases. Ann Thorac Surg 1991;51(2):219–24.
94. Canter RJ, Qin LX, Downey RJ, et al. Perioperative chemotherapy in patients undergoing pulmonary resection for metastatic soft-tissue sarcoma of the extremity: a retrospective analysis. Cancer 2007;110(9):2050–60.
95. Liapi E, Geschwind JF. Transcatheter and ablative therapeutic approaches for solid malignancies. J Clin Oncol 2007;25(8):978–86.
96. Nakamura T, Matsumine A, Yamakado K, et al. Lung radiofrequency ablation in patients with pulmonary metastases from musculoskeletal sarcomas [corrected]. Cancer 2009;115(16):3774–81.
97. Ketchedjian A, Daly B, Luketich J, et al. Minimally invasive techniques for managing pulmonary metastases: video-assisted thoracic surgery and radiofrequency ablation. Thorac Surg Clin 2006;16(2):157–65.
98. Siva S, MacManus M, Ball D. Stereotactic radiotherapy for pulmonary oligometastases: a systematic review. J Thorac Oncol 2010;5(7):1091–9.

99. Dhakal S, Corbin KS, Milano MT, et al. Stereotactic body radiotherapy for pulmonary metastases from soft-tissue sarcomas: excellent local lesion control and improved patient survival. Int J Radiat Oncol Biol Phys 2011 [Epub ahead of print].
100. Casson AG, Putnam JB, Natarajan G, et al. Efficacy of pulmonary metastasectomy for recurrent soft tissue sarcoma. J Surg Oncol 1991;47(1):1–4.
101. Rizzoni WE, Pass HI, Wesley MN, et al. Resection of recurrent pulmonary metastases in patients with soft-tissue sarcomas. Arch Surg 1986;121(11):1248–52.

Isolated Regional Therapy for Advanced Extremity Soft Tissue Sarcomas

Jeremiah L. Deneve, DO[a], Jonathan S. Zager, MD[a,b,c],*

KEYWORDS

- Sarcoma • Isolated limb infusion
- Hyperthermic isolated limb perfusion • Regional perfusion
- Wieberdink scale

Patients with large, locally advanced soft tissue sarcoma (STS) of the extremities represent a small percentage of adult malignancies and have a high risk of local recurrence and distant metastasis. Obtaining adequate local control may require radical, functionally debilitating surgery, which could have a profound impact on limb function and the patient's quality of life. Amputation of the affected extremity may provide durable local control,[1] but at the expense of loss of function and without an improvement in overall outcome.[2] For patients with STS who present with unresectable bulky primary tumors or recurrent tumors with distant disease, selecting the most appropriate treatment that allows patients to maintain function without compromising quality of life, limb function, and long-term outcomes is a challenge.

Over the past few decades, there has been a growing trend toward limb-preservation therapies when treating patients with unresectable, recurrent or bulky, locally advanced primary STS tumors. Offering the potential for limb salvage by treating the local or regional disease process without compromising extremity function ultimately may allow patients to maintain a better quality of life while avoiding the need for amputation. Regional delivery of chemotherapy addresses these concerns and can be used as a potential adjunct to surgical resection with radiation therapy for advanced

This work was not supported by any commercial funding.
The authors have nothing to disclose.
[a] Cutaneous Oncology Department, Moffitt Cancer Center, 12902 Magnolia Drive, SRB4. 24016, Tampa, FL 33612, USA
[b] Department of Oncologic Sciences, University of South Florida, 12902 Magnolia Drive, SRB4. 24012, Tampa, FL 33612, USA
[c] Department of Surgery, University of South Florida, 12902 Magnolia Drive, SRB4. 24012, Tampa, FL 33612, USA
* Corresponding author. Department of Oncologic Sciences, University of South Florida, 12902 Magnolia Drive, SRB4. 24012, Tampa, FL 33612.
E-mail address: Jonathan.Zager@Moffitt.org

extremity STS tumors previously deemed unresectable. Two techniques, hyper-thermic isolated limb perfusion (HILP) and isolated limb infusion (ILI), allow the regional administration of chemotherapy, delivering drug concentrations 15 to 25 times higher than systemic dosages without the systemic side effects.[3] For patients with advanced, unresectable STS with limited treatment options, both procedures are well tolerated, repeatable (especially in the case of ILI), and have acceptable toxicity profiles. This article describes the role of HILP and ILI in the management of patients with advanced, limb-threatening extremity STS.

INDICATIONS FOR REGIONAL THERAPY

Patients who are referred to centers that specialize in regional therapies have often been maximally treated with one or more previous surgical operations or have received adjuvant radiation treatment or chemotherapy. For those patients who relapse, many are deemed "unresectable" based on involvement of critical structures, such as neurovascular bundles, or have developed distant disease. Others may present with primary tumors that are potentially marginally resectable, but after radical surgery and adjuvant radiation treatment would be disfigured or left with a functionally impaired extremity. For these reasons, many patients in these situations are referred for ultimate local control by extremity amputation. Unfortunately, amputation confers no long-term survival benefit over limb-sparing.[4,5] However, these patients may be the ideal candidates for regional therapy with HILP or ILI.

The indications for regional therapy are numerous, most importantly those patients with unresectable, extremity STS or those in whom resection would result in a disfig-ured or severely functionally impaired limb. Other indications include multifocal primary tumors,[6] recurrent disease,[7] prior resection with irradiation,[8] bulky primary tumor size,[9–11] or high-grade tumors.[9] Elderly patients[12] and those treated in the palli-ative setting also have been shown to gain a benefit in local control and limb salvage rates with regional therapy.[11] Finally, other less frequently encountered noncutaneous and STS types have also been described in the literature to be amenable to regional chemoperfusion therapy including Kaposi sarcoma,[13] Stewart-Treves lymphangiosar-coma,[14,15] desmoid tumors,[9,14] Merkel cell carcinoma,[16,17] and osteosarcoma.[18]

TECHNIQUE OF HILP

First reported in the 1950s for treating melanoma patients with regional disease,[3] HILP was the first established therapy to gain acceptance for regional chemoperfusion to improve limb salvage rates in patients with extremity STS. The technique has been extensively described in the literature.[19] Briefly, HILP requires surgical exposure and cannulation of the iliac or femoral vessels for lower-extremity tumors or subclavian or axillary vessels for upper-extremity tumors. Cannulae are connected to an extracor-poreal circuit that contains a membrane oxygenator and heat exchanger. The circuit is primed with blood, Ringer's lactate solution, and heparin. To ensure complete vascular isolation and target tumor perfusion, a pneumatic cuff or Esmark tourniquet is applied proximally on the affected extremity. Systemic leakage is measured contin-uously during the procedure by a precordial Geiger counter that monitors ^{99}Tc radio-labled human serum albumin or red blood cells previously injected into the perfusate. Flow rates are set as high as possible, generally 35 to 40 mL/L of limb volume per minute, and are adjusted based on the percentage of leakage. The procedure is per-formed under hyperthermic conditions (38.5–40°C). After the desired limb temperature is reached and there is no evidence of systemic leakage (<0.5%), the intended chemo-therapeutic regimen is administered.

Melphalan is the drug of choice for HILP and dosage is calculated according to the liter-volume method.[20] Although several different cytotoxic regimens have been investigated for use in regional therapy for extremity STS, including cisplatin[21] and dacarbazine,[22] none have exceeded the outcomes observed using melphalan.[23] Actinomycin D, when used in combination with melphalan, has shown favorable response rates[24] and is currently the regimen used for ILI regional therapy in many centers in the United States. European centers initially used a three-drug regimen with recombinant tumor necrosis factor (TNF)-α (2–4 mg), recombinant interferon (IFN)-γ (0.2 mg), and melphalan (10 mg/L for lower limb and 13 mg/L for upper limb) when treating advanced melanoma and patients with STS with HILP.[7] However, early results showed that most of the tumor-related response was TNF-α–related and INF-γ use was subsequently abandoned.[9,10,25,26]

The perfusion is performed for a total of 90 minutes. At the completion of the procedure, the limb is flushed with 2 to 4 L of isotonic saline solution, tourniquets are released, and vascular anatomy is reconstructed. Postoperatively, patients are observed in an intensive care setting for hydration and monitoring for systemic toxicity and reperfusion injury. Average postoperative hospital length of stay ranges from 8 to 10 days.

TECHNIQUE OF ILI

ILI, a less invasive approach for administering regional chemotherapy, was developed and first reported on by the Sydney Melanoma Unit.[27] Initially described for the treatment of in-transit metastases in melanoma patients, ILI is a less complex, less invasive procedure that has been shown to have overall response rates close to those observed after conventional HILP. ILI is essentially a low-flow HILP performed under hyperthermic, nonoxygenated conditions by percutaneously placed catheters. ILI was first described in patients with advanced extremity STS using doxorubicin (0.7 mg/kg upper limb, 1.4 mg/kg lower limb) in conjunction with preoperative radiotherapy and delayed surgical resection with the aim of improving limb preservation.[6] Since that time, several other institutions have reported on their experience using ILI for advanced extremity STS.[17,28–30]

On the day of the procedure, high-flow 5F to 6F arterial and 6F to 8F venous catheters are inserted by way of the uninvolved lower extremity (femoral artery and vein, respectively) using the Seldinger technique and advanced under fluoroscopic guidance into the involved extremity. After the induction of general anesthesia, heparin is given to achieve full systemic anticoagulation with a target activated clotting time greater than or equal to 350 seconds. The arterial and venous catheters are then connected to an infusion circuit that consists of a heat exchanger and bubble excluder. After subcutaneous temperatures of greater than 37°C are achieved, a pneumatic tourniquet (inflated to 250–300) or an Esmark wrap is placed on the proximal aspect of the limb to be infused, isolating the limb from the systemic circulation. Papaverine (60 mg) is injected into the arterial catheter and chemoperfusion is initiated. Depending on the chemotherapeutic regimen used (frequently actinomycin D and melphalan), cytotoxic agents are typically circulated for 30 minutes. After 30 minutes of infusion, the limb is manually flushed with 750 to 1000 mL of isotonic crystalloid solution. After the washout period, the tourniquet is removed, heparinization is reversed with protamine if necessary, and the catheters are removed when the activated clotting time is at or near baseline. Patients are monitored daily for regional toxicity with serial creatine phosphokinase (CPK) measurements and are discharged home when CPK levels peak and then fall back toward the baseline, generally within 4 to 6 days.[17]

TOXICITY

The toxicity profile for HILP and ILI is described in acute and long-term side effects and is further classified as either systemic or regional toxicities.[31] In general, the toxicity of HILP is more severe than that experienced by patients who undergo ILI procedures.

Systemic Toxicity After HILP or ILI

Systemic toxicities, in particular, are seen more frequently with HILP procedures and are related to the type of chemotherapy used and amount of leakage of the chemotherapeutic into the systemic circulation. Leakage rates less than 3% to 4% are generally well tolerated. However, higher flow rates may result in increased systemic leakage, producing gastrointestinal, hematopoietic, or other constitutional side effects.[32] Continuous precordial monitoring for systemic leakage is mandatory for patients undergoing HILP therapy. To minimize potential systemic toxicity post-HILP, some authors have suggested that prolonged washout during the termination portion of the perfusion may also further help reduce systemic toxicity complications.[33]

The potential systemic toxicities described after HILP include the hematologic, gastrointestinal, genitourinary, cardiac, pulmonary, neurologic, and integumentary systems.[34] TNF-α, which is commonly used in many European centers, is thought to be responsible for many of the systemic toxicities experienced with HILP. TNF-α targets tumor microvasculature, which results in coagulative and hemorrhagic necrosis of tumors.[35] Systemic leakage of TNF-α can induce a severe systemic inflammatory response syndrome with hypotension and shock-like symptoms, which necessitates aggressive hydration and vasopressor resuscitation. Eggermont and colleagues,[9] in a multicenter HILP trial treating 186 patients with locally advanced extremity STS using TNF-α and melphalan, found only a mild to moderate systemic toxicity profile attributable to high-dose TNF-α (2–4 mg). This was easily managed and associated with no toxicity-related deaths. Most patients had mild fever or chills, controlled with antipyretics. Only 3% of patients developed grades III to IV cardiovascular toxicity, managed with vasopressor agents and hydration. In another report of 217 HILP procedures using TNF-α and melphalan for limb-threatening STS, there were minimal sequelae for patients with leak rates less than 10% (88% of patients).[14] Six patients had leak rates greater than 20%. Their procedures were subsequently terminated, but none went on to develop severe complication or require intensive care unit monitoring for more than 24 hours. These results suggest that appropriate monitoring and supportive care may offset much of the TNF-α–induced toxicity without significant long-term sequelae.

Systemic toxicity related to ILI is much less common than that experienced after HILP. Early reports of ILI in advanced extremity STS noted no specific systemic toxicity.[6] Symptoms experienced by most patients are mild (eg, nausea) and self-limiting, often resolving by postoperative Days 1 or 2.[28,36] Rhabdomyolysis, as measured by serum CPK, is commonly encountered in patients undergoing this form of regional therapy. CPK levels often rise greater than 1000 IU/L and require daily blood urea nitrogen and creatinine level monitoring to avoid myoglobin-induced renal failure. Aggressive hydration with isotonic saline, maintaining a urine output of greater than 0.5 mL/kg/h, may reduce the risk of renal failure caused by myoglobinuria.[27,36,37] Patients with CPK levels greater than 1000 IU/L are hydrated, given corticosteroids to decrease muscle edema or inflammation, and monitored until CPK levels have peaked and fallen less than 1000 IU/L. In a multicenter report of 12 patients with locally advanced STS undergoing ILI, CPK levels peaked around Day 3 with median levels of 127 for the upper extremity and 93 for the lower extremity. No patient developed any short- or long-term sequelae because of CPK-related toxicity.[17]

Regional Toxicity After HILP or ILI

Regional toxicity after HILP or ILI is common and results in short- and long-term morbidity. A commonly used classification system characterizing acute tissue reactions after HILP or ILI was first reported by Wieberdink and colleagues.[20] Briefly, it characterizes acute regional toxicity on a one to five scale with grade I toxicity representing no injury. Grade II toxicity is described as a soft tissue reaction manifesting as slight erythema or edema of the extremity. Grade III toxicity consist of considerable erythema or edema with some blistering. Grade IV injury involves extensive epidermolysis, which may cause definite functional disturbance with the threat or manifestation of compartment syndrome requiring fasciotomy. Grade V toxicity is characterized by severe tissue necrosis or vascular catastrophe that results in amputation. This classification system has standardized regional toxicity reporting for patients undergoing HILP or ILI therapy (**Table 1**).

Acute regional toxicity-related symptoms are seen within the first 48 hours after HILP or 72 to 96 hours after ILI.[27,37,38] Typical reactions to therapy are mild erythema, edema, and pain (Wieberdink grades II–III). Mild or moderate blistering is not uncommon and is seen up to several days posttherapy. Mild erythema or edema, when present, may persist for months after treatment. Other acute complications including vascular injury, thrombosis, compartment syndrome, and tissue loss leading to amputation have also been reported.[26,39–42] In the first description of ILI therapy for limb-threatening STS, no significant regional toxicity-related complications were reported.[6] Forty patients underwent preoperative ILI with doxorubicin followed by external-beam radiation and delayed resection. Only 30% of patients experience grades II or III toxicity. In a multicenter study of ILI for nonmelanoma cutaneous and STS malignancies, Turaga and colleagues[17] reported on 22 patients undergoing 26 ILI treatments with melphalan and D-actinomycin over a 5-year period. Most patients (96%) had grade III toxicity or less; only one (4%) developed grade IV toxicity. The authors concluded that ILI offers good extremity function preservation with only minimal morbidity.

Long-term regional toxicity is less frequently reported for patients undergoing regional therapy with HILP. In the largest HILP multicenter experience for STS to date, most patients (92%) had mild perfusion reaction (grades II and III), whereas 14 patients experienced grade IV toxicity.[9] The authors noted that 20% developed transient distal extremity paresthesias, whereas 3% developed long-term peroneal

Table 1 Wieberdink toxicity scale	
Grade	**Clinical Characteristics**
I	No subjective or objective evidence of reaction
II	Slight erythema or edema
III	Considerable erythema or edema with some blistering; slightly disturbed motility permissible
IV	Extensive epidermolysis or obvious damage to the deep tissues causing definite functional disturbances; threatened or manifest compartmental syndromes
V	Reaction that may necessitate amputation

nerve dysfunction. Similar findings were reported in 49 patients undergoing HILP with TNF-α and melphalan for unresectable STS; short- and long-term complications were described in detail.[26] Most patients (71%) had mild acute regional toxicity (grade II). Three patients (6%) developed major complications after ILP: two patients developed arterial thrombosis treated with thrombectomy, another developed a life-threatening clostridial wound infection and died 2 days after ILP. Long-term functional morbidity was also described: 31% had some sort of extremity malfunction 1 year post-HILP, whereas four patients suffered permanent nerve dysfunction.

OUTCOME AFTER HILP FOR EXTREMITY STS

In one of the earliest reports of regional therapy for STS, Lienard and colleagues[7] performed 25 HILPs in 23 patients with advanced melanoma or STS (N = 4). Using a multidrug regimen of high-dose TNF-α (2–4 mg), IFN-γ (0.2 mg), and melphalan (10 mg/L for lower limb, 13 mg/L for upper limb), 21 patients (89%) developed a complete response (CR) and 2 had a partial response (PR), essentially no treatment failures. Overall survival was 76% at 12 months of follow-up. Although most patients in this study were treated for advanced melanoma, these findings confirmed the proof of concept for the successful treatment of recurrent STS using regional therapy while avoiding amputation with acceptable outcomes. This early work was later supplanted by a larger multicenter European HILP trial treating specifically patients with nonresectable extremity STS.[43] Fifty-five patients with primary (N = 30) or recurrent (N = 25) STS were treated with HILP using a similar multichemotherapeutic regimen. The clinical CR rate, as defined by gross tumor disappearance, was 18%; a clinical PR rate of 64% and no change was observed in 18%. When determined by the clinical and pathologic response to treatment, outcomes were much better: 36% CR, 51% PR, and 13% no change, respectively.

Although these initial experiences showed promising results, additional studies using melphalan with TNF-α formed the foundation for the role of regional therapy in patients with advanced extremity STS previously only considered for amputation. Tumor response rates ranging from 68% to 91% have been reported from several centers using TNF-α and melphalan[9,10,14,26] irrespective of the dose of TNF-α used.[44] From the largest reported series of HILPs in patients with limb-threatening STS, Grunhagen and colleagues[14] noted a 75% overall response rate (CR in 26% and PR of 49%). Rossi and colleagues,[45] investigating the combination of other cyto-toxic agents with TNF-α, reported on their experience with HILP using doxorubicin (8.5 mg/L limb volume) for patients with limb-threatening STS. Doxorubicin, an active anti-blastic agent, was found to be synergistic with low-dose TNF-α (1 mg) in early phase I and II study by the same authors.[46,47] Building on their prior experience, a major histo-logic response for doxorubicin–TNF-α was identified in 90% of 21 patients treated. Clinical responses were 5% CR and 57% PR. Although several cytotoxic combinations have been studied to optimize tumor response rates with HILP, TNF-α with melphalan remains the most frequently used regimen at many European centers.

OUTCOME AFTER ILI FOR EXTREMITY STS

Early experience with ILI therapy for limb-threatening STS has also produced encouraging results comparable with those for patients undergoing HILP. In 2007, the first description of regional therapy using ILI for STS (as neoadjuvant treatment with surgery and radiation treatment) was from Hegazy and colleagues.[6] Forty patients underwent preoperative ILI with doxorubicin (0.7 mg/kg for upper limbs, 1.4 mg/kg for lower limbs) followed by external-beam radiotherapy (37 Gy) 3 to 7 days after ILI. Patients were then taken for limb-preserving resection 3 to 7 weeks after initial treatment. Results were promising with tumor responses observed in 85% of patients, rendering most patients resectable. With a median follow-up of 15 months, only four patients (13%) recurred locally; two were managed with reresection, one with amputation, and one with chemotherapy. The Sydney Melanoma Unit, the original developers of ILI, reported on their initial ILI experience for locally advanced STS in 2008.[29] Twenty-one patients were treated, 14 (67%) as neoadjuvant therapy before surgery and 7 (33%) for inoperable recurrence or palliation. Using primarily actinomycin D (50–100 µg/L) and melphalan (5–10 mg/L), an overall tumor response of 90% was obtained (57% CR and 33% PR). Patients with a CR had significantly lower local recurrence rates, which, along with MFH subtype, were identified as an independent predictor of local recurrence. At a median follow-up of 28 months, overall disease-specific survival was 62% with stages III and IV disease having worse survival. There were similar findings from a United States multicenter collaborative effort using ILI for locally advanced nonmelanoma cutaneous malignancies by Turaga and colleagues.[17] Twenty-two patients (12 with STS) underwent treatment using melphalan and actinomycin D. For the patients with STS, all had undergone prior maximal therapy with surgical resection or radiation treatment and had been referred for amputation. The 12 patients with STS underwent 14 ILI procedures. With a median follow-up of 11 months, the overall tumor response was 78% (14% CR, 64% PR) per ILI performed. The overall 3-month in-field response rate was 79% (21% CR, 58% PR) for all patients treated in this study. Although few studies have been published on ILI for STS, work by several centers has revealed promising results and will continue to be the focus of future collaboration and research.

LIMB PRESERVATION WITH HILP

Historically, varying treatment strategies have been used to improve limb salvage rates, including neoadjuvant chemotherapy,[48] preoperative radiation therapy,[49] and marginal resection with brachytherapy.[50] Using HILP for advanced extremity STS, limb preservation rates have been consistently reported to range from 57% to 87%.[9,11,14,26]

Grunhagen and colleagues[14] treated 197 patients with 217 consecutive HILP procedures using TNF-α and melphalan. The limb salvage rate was 87%. Twenty-six patients (13%) required amputation, 15 for no response to HILP, 9 for rapid progression of disease, and 2 delayed amputations for preexisting vascular disease. Other authors using high-dose TNF-α and melphalan have noted similar limb-preservations rates. In the multicenter European experience of HILP therapy in 186 patients with STS, Eggermont and colleagues[9] observed an 82% limb salvage rate. Thirty-four patients (18%) required amputation, most for disease progression or recurrence. Three patients who had a CR after HILP required amputation for wound healing issues, two of whom had prior radiation treatment. In a similar experience treating 22 patients with 24 HILPs using TNF-α and melphalan, Lejeune and colleagues[25] found 86% limb salvage rate with only three patients (14%) requiring amputation. One patient required amputation after a second HILP procedure for no response. Two patients required late amputation for progression with diffuse recurrence. Gutman and colleagues[10] reported a greater than 90% response rate and 85% limb-preservation rate in 35 patients who underwent 41 HILPs. Five patients (14%) underwent amputation, three for no response to HILP, one for disease progression after resection of a tumor involving the nerve bundle, and one for uncontrolled sepsis.

The combination of radiotherapy in the adjuvant and neoadjuvant setting with HILP for STS has also been investigated. Olieman and colleagues[11] reported on the efficacy of adjuvant radiation treatment after HILP with TNF-α, IFN-γ, and melphalan and delayed surgical resection. Of 34 patients treated, limb salvage was achieved in 29 patients (85%): 14 patients with HILP plus radiotherapy and 15 patients after only HILP. Five patients required amputation, which was performed from 5 days to 6 weeks, for radiation-induced necrosis (N = 1), progressive local disease (N = 2), and treatment-related complications (N = 2). The authors concluded that adjuvant radiotherapy after HILP and marginal resection increased local control without compounding radiation-induced morbidity. Lans and colleagues[51] reported on 30 HILP performed for recurrent STS in 26 patients who had previously been resected and irradiated. Eleven patients presented with multifocal tumor and all patients were being considered for amputation. The affected extremity was successfully preserved in 17 patients (65%). Nine patients recurred, five of whom underwent amputation to achieve local control. The remainder underwent delayed resection or was managed expectantly because of distant disease. These authors concluded that patients with recurrence who have been previously resected and irradiated should be considered for HILP therapy as an alternative to amputation.

LIMB PRESERVATION WITH ILI

ILI also offers an acceptable and attractive limb-sparing alternative to amputation for extremity STS recurrence. ILI in patients with advanced STS has produced limb-preservation rates equal to those reported with HILP and without many of the toxicity-related side effects. Hegazy and colleagues[6] first reported on 40 patients with unresectable extremity STS who underwent ILI using doxorubicin followed by external-beam radiotherapy and then delayed resection. All patients in this study were initially considered for amputation. A clinical tumor response was achieved in 85% of patients. Three patients underwent amputation for a limb-salvage rate of 82.5%. The Sydney Melanoma Unit reported on 21 patients who underwent ILI over a 13-year period, primarily using melphalan and actinomycin D.[29] A 90% overall response rate was achieved, 100% for patients undergoing ILI as neoadjuvant therapy before surgical resection. Amputation for disease progression was necessary in only five patients for an overall limb salvage rate of 76%. Similar limb-preservation rates were noted by Turaga and colleagues.[17] Twenty-two patients underwent 26 ILI procedures during a 5-year period. The primary end points of this study were limb preservation and in-field response rates. All patients had previously failed maximal limb-salvage treatment with surgery and radiation treatment and were considered for amputation. Successful limb preservation was achievable in 19 (86%) of the 22 patients for all patients treated and 78% for the 12 patients with STS. The authors concluded that the role of ILI could possibly be expanded to include neoadjuvant use, which may allow surgical resection in these patients and maintain extremity function while avoiding amputation, although it should be done in a clinical trial setting. A brief summary of the treatment and outcome data in patients with advanced extremity STS who undergo regional therapy is listed in **Table 2**.

PALLIATIVE ISOLATED REGIONAL THERAPY

In the setting of widespread metastases, the local disease process can be a significant source of discomfort and frustration for patients with STS and their clinicians. Improving local disease control with regional therapy, whether for curative or palliative purposes, may address these concerns and offer a better quality of life for patients

Table 2
Treatment and outcome data for all patients undergoing regional therapy for advanced extremity soft tissue sarcoma

Investigator	Year	N	Modality	Chemo in Perfusate	Median Follow-up (mo)	ORR (%)	CR/PR/SD (%)	Limb Preservation (%)
Eggermont et al[9]	1996	186	HILP	TNF-α IFN-γ (N = 55) Melphalan	22	82	29/53/18	82
Eggermont et al[43]	1996	55	HILP	TNF-α IFN-γ Melphalan	26	87	36/51/13	84
Gutman et al[10]	1997	35	HILP	TNF-α Melphalan	14	91	37/54/8.5	85
Olieman et al[11]	1998	34	HILP	TNF-α IFN-γ Melphalan	34	94	35/59/6	85
Lejeune et al[25]	2000	22	HILP	TNF-α IFN-γ (N = 4) Melphalan	18.7	82	18/64/18	86
Noorda et al[26]	2003	49	HILP	TNF-α, IFN-γ (N = 4) Melphalan	26	63	8/55/35	57
Rossi et al[53]	2005	21	HILP	TNF-α Doxorubicin	30	62	5/57/38	71
Grunhagen et al[8]	2005	53	HILP	TNF-α Melphalan	22	88	42/45/13	82
Bonvalot et al[44]	2005	100	HILP	TNF-α Melphalan	24	65	36/29/35	87
Lans et al[53]	2005	26	HILP	TNF-α Melphalan	22	70	20/50/30	65
Grunhagen et al[14]	2006	197	HILP	TNF-α Melphalan	22	75	26/49/25	87
Hegazy et al[6]	2007	40	ILI	Doxorubicin	15	85	—/85/—	83
Moncrieff et al[29]	2008	21	ILI	Melphalan Actin D	28	90	57/33/10	76
Turaga et al[17]	2011	12	ILI	Melphalan Actin D	8.6	78	14/64/—	78

Abbreviations: Actin D, actinomycin D; N, patients treated; ORR, overall response rate; SD, no change or progression of disease.

with a historically limited lifespan. In one of the largest multicenter HILP reports to date, 13% of patients with known distant disease underwent HILP for palliative purposes.[9] Limb salvage was achieved in 92%. Olieman and colleagues[52] reported on the palliative use of limb-salvage HILP for patients with STS with known regional or distant metastases. Nine patients underwent regional therapy with a median follow-up of 9 months. Limb preservation was possible in 89% with only one patient experiencing limb failure requiring amputation. Certainly, regional therapy may be a suitable limb-salvage alternative to amputation for patients who present with locally advanced disease in the setting of distant metastases.

LOCOREGIONAL RECURRENCE AFTER ISOLATED REGIONAL THERAPY

Local or regional recurrence after HILP as reported in the literature varies between 11% and 48%.[9–11,25] Eggermont and colleagues[43] noted 10 local recurrences (18%) in 55 patients treated for nonresectable extremity STS. For the subset of patients with multifocal tumors treated with HILP, the recurrence rate was 38%. Alternatively, in patients able to undergo resection after HILP, the local recurrence rate was low at 13%. Three patients subsequently underwent multiple perfusions, one after an initial PR and another after progressive disease. The third patient had a total of three HILP performed for more than 100 tumors involving the upper extremity.

Similar recurrence rates of 13% to 42% have also been reported for patients with STS undergoing ILI.[6,29] In the Sydney Melanoma Unit experience, 9 patients (42%) recurred out of 21 patients treated.[29] For patients who were able to successfully undergo surgical resection of their tumor after ILI, the recurrence rate was only 21%. Therefore, surgical resection after ILI was associated with a significant decrease in local recurrence. No patient underwent repeat ILI for recurrence in that series. In contrast, Turaga and colleagues[17] managed their patients with STS recurrence after initial ILI using repeated ILI therapy. Two out of 12 patients with STS in that series, both with an initial response to ILI, underwent repeated ILI for relapse. Consequently, for patients who recur after prior isolated regional therapy, repeat regional therapy by HILP or ILI is a reasonable treatment alternative to amputation, even in the presence of distant metastases.

SUMMARY

Patients who present with unresectable, large, primary or recurrent extremity STS or locally advanced tumors in the setting of systemic disease have effective treatment options available in the form of isolated regional therapies. HILP and ILI have proved to be efficacious with acceptable systemic and regional toxicity profiles. Both procedures are repeatable (especially ILI) and are an attractive option as either definitive treatment or as neoadjuvant therapy combined with surgery and radiation treatment for patients with advanced, maximally treated, or unresectable extremity STS. ILI is an exciting and continued area of interest as more centers gain familiarity with its use. Ongoing multicenter collaborations and clinical trials are required as clinicians continue to gain knowledge on regional therapy and expand the indications for its use in the management of advanced extremity STS.

REFERENCES

1. Pisters PW, Leung DH, Woodruff J, et al. Analysis of prognostic factors in 1,041 patients with localized soft tissue sarcomas of the extremities. J Clin Oncol 1996;14:1679–89.
2. Williard WC, Collin C, Casper ES, et al. The changing role of amputation for soft tissue sarcoma of the extremity in adults. Surg Gynecol Obstet 1992;175: 389–96.
3. Creech O Jr, Krementz ET, Ryan RF, et al. Chemotherapy of cancer: regional perfusion utilizing an extracorporeal circuit. Ann Surg 1958;148:616–32.
4. Collin CF, Friedrich C, Godbold J, et al. Prognostic factors for local recurrence and survival in patients with localized extremity soft-tissue sarcoma. Semin Surg Oncol 1988;4:30–7.
5. Collin C, Godbold J, Hajdu S, et al. Localized extremity soft tissue sarcoma: an analysis of factors affecting survival. J Clin Oncol 1987;5:601–12.

6. Hegazy MA, Kotb SZ, Sakr H, et al. Preoperative isolated limb infusion of doxorubicin and external irradiation for limb-threatening soft tissue sarcomas. Ann Surg Oncol 2007;14:568–76.
7. Lienard D, Ewalenko P, Delmotte JJ, et al. High-dose recombinant tumor necrosis factor alpha in combination with interferon gamma and melphalan in isolation perfusion of the limbs for melanoma and sarcoma. J Clin Oncol 1992;10:52–60.
8. Grunhagen DJ, Brunstein F, Graveland WJ, et al. Isolated limb perfusion with tumor necrosis factor and melphalan prevents amputation in patients with multiple sarcomas in arm or leg. Ann Surg Oncol 2005;12:473–9.
9. Eggermont AM, Schraffordt Koops H, Klausner JM, et al. Isolated limb perfusion with tumor necrosis factor and melphalan for limb salvage in 186 patients with locally advanced soft tissue extremity sarcomas. The cumulative multicenter European experience. Ann Surg 1996;224:756–64 [discussion: 764–5].
10. Gutman M, Inbar M, Lev-Shlush D, et al. High dose tumor necrosis factor-alpha and melphalan administered via isolated limb perfusion for advanced limb soft tissue sarcoma results in a >90% response rate and limb preservation. Cancer 1997;79:1129–37.
11. Olieman AF, Pras E, van Ginkel RJ, et al. Feasibility and efficacy of external beam radiotherapy after hyperthermic isolated limb perfusion with TNF-alpha and melphalan for limb-saving treatment in locally advanced extremity soft-tissue sarcoma. Int J Radiat Oncol Biol Phys 1998;40:807–14.
12. van Etten B, van Geel AN, de Wilt JH, et al. Fifty tumor necrosis factor-based isolated limb perfusions for limb salvage in patients older than 75 years with limb-threatening soft tissue sarcomas and other extremity tumors. Ann Surg Oncol 2003;10:32–7.
13. Lev-Chelouche D, Abu-Abeid S, Merimsky O, et al. Isolated limb perfusion with high-dose tumor necrosis factor alpha and melphalan for Kaposi sarcoma. Arch Surg 1999;134:177–80.
14. Grunhagen DJ, de Wilt JH, Graveland WJ, et al. Outcome and prognostic factor analysis of 217 consecutive isolated limb perfusions with tumor necrosis factor-alpha and melphalan for limb-threatening soft tissue sarcoma. Cancer 2006;106:1776–84.
15. Lans TE, de Wilt JH, van Geel AN, et al. Isolated limb perfusion with tumor necrosis factor and melphalan for nonresectable Stewart-Treves lymphangiosarcoma. Ann Surg Oncol 2002;9:1004–9.
16. Olieman AF, Lienard D, Eggermont AM, et al. Hyperthermic isolated limb perfusion with tumor necrosis factor alpha, interferon gamma, and melphalan for locally advanced nonmelanoma skin tumors of the extremities: a multicenter study. Arch Surg 1999;134:303–7.
17. Turaga KK, Beasley GM, Kane JMIII, et al. Limb preservation with isolated limb infusion for locally advanced nonmelanoma cutaneous and soft-tissue malignant neoplasms. Arch Surg 2011;146:870–5.
18. Bickels J, Manusama ER, Gutman M, et al. Isolated limb perfusion with tumour necrosis factor-alpha and melphalan for unresectable bone sarcomas of the lower extremity. Eur J Surg Oncol 1999;25:509–14.
19. Lejeune FJ, Ghanem GE. A simple and accurate new method for cytostatics dosimetry in isolation perfusion of the limbs based on exchangeable blood volume determination. Cancer Res 1987;47:639–43.
20. Wieberdink J, Benckhuysen C, Braat RP, et al. Dosimetry in isolation perfusion of the limbs by assessment of perfused tissue volume and grading of toxic tissue reactions. Eur J Cancer Clin Oncol 1982;18:905–10.

21. Hoekstra HJ, Schraffordt Koops H, de Vries LG, et al. Toxicity of hyperthermic isolated limb perfusion with cisplatin for recurrent melanoma of the lower extremity after previous perfusion treatment. Cancer 1993;72:1224–9.

22. Bonenkamp JJ, Thompson JF, de Wilt JH, et al. Isolated limb infusion with fotemustine after dacarbazine chemosensitisation for inoperable loco-regional melanoma recurrence. Eur J Surg Oncol 2004;30:1107–12.

23. Briele HA, Djuric M, Jung DT, et al. Pharmacokinetics of melphalan in clinical isolation perfusion of the extremities. Cancer Res 1985;45:1885–9.

24. Thompson JF, Hunt JA, Shannon KF, et al. Frequency and duration of remission after isolated limb perfusion for melanoma. Arch Surg 1997;132:903–7.

25. Lejeune FJ, Pujol N, Lienard D, et al. Limb salvage by neoadjuvant isolated perfusion with TNF alpha and melphalan for non-resectable soft tissue sarcoma of the extremities. Eur J Surg Oncol 2000;26:669–78.

26. Noorda EM, Vrouenraets BC, Nieweg OE, et al. Isolated limb perfusion with tumor necrosis factor-alpha and melphalan for patients with unresectable soft tissue sarcoma of the extremities. Cancer 2003;98:1483–90.

27. Thompson JF, Kam PC, Waugh RC, et al. Isolated limb infusion with cytotoxic agents: a simple alternative to isolated limb perfusion. Semin Surg Oncol 1998;14:238–47.

28. Brady MS, Brown K, Patel A, et al. Isolated limb infusion with melphalan and dactinomycin for regional melanoma and soft-tissue sarcoma of the extremity: final report of a phase II clinical trial. Melanoma Res 2009;19:106–11.

29. Moncrieff MD, Kroon HM, Kam PC, et al. Isolated limb infusion for advanced soft tissue sarcoma of the extremity. Ann Surg Oncol 2008;15:2749–56.

30. Brady MS, Brown K, Patel A, et al. A phase II trial of isolated limb infusion with melphalan and dactinomycin for regional melanoma and soft tissue sarcoma of the extremity. Ann Surg Oncol 2006;13:1123–9.

31. Moller MG, Lewis JM, Dessureault S, et al. Toxicities associated with hyperthermic isolated limb perfusion and isolated limb infusion in the treatment of melanoma and sarcoma. Int J Hyperthermia 2008;24:275–89.

32. Sorkin P, Abu-Abid S, Lev D, et al. Systemic leakage and side effects of tumor necrosis factor alpha administered via isolated limb perfusion can be manipulated by flow rate adjustment. Arch Surg 1995;130:1079–84.

33. Lienard D, Eggermont AM, Schraffordt Koops H, et al. Isolated perfusion of the limb with high-dose tumour necrosis factor-alpha (TNF-alpha), interferon-gamma (IFN-gamma) and melphalan for melanoma stage III. Results of a multicentre pilot study. Melanoma Res 1994;(Suppl 1):21–6.

34. Miller AB, Hoogstraten B, Staquet M, et al. Reporting results of cancer treatment. Cancer 1981;47:207–14.

35. Renard N, Lienard D, Lespagnard L, et al. Early endothelium activation and polymorphonuclear cell invasion precede specific necrosis of human melanoma and sarcoma treated by intravascular high-dose tumour necrosis factor alpha (rTNF alpha). Int J Cancer 1994;57:656–63.

36. Santillan AA, Delman KA, Beasley GM, et al. Predictive factors of regional toxicity and serum creatine phosphokinase levels after isolated limb infusion for melanoma: a multi-institutional analysis. Ann Surg Oncol 2009;16:2570–8.

37. Thompson JF, Kam PC. Isolated limb infusion for melanoma: a simple but effective alternative to isolated limb perfusion. J Surg Oncol 2004;88:1–3.

38. Vrouenraets BC, Klaase JM, Nieweg OE, et al. Toxicity and morbidity of isolated limb perfusion. Semin Surg Oncol 1998;14:224–31.

39. Cornett WR, McCall LM, Petersen RP, et al. Randomized multicenter trial of hyperthermic isolated limb perfusion with melphalan alone compared with melphalan

plus tumor necrosis factor: American College of Surgeons Oncology Group Trial Z0020. J Clin Oncol 2006;24:4196–201.

40. Eroglu A, Ozcan H, Eryavuz Y, et al. Deep venous thrombosis of the extremity diagnosed by color Doppler ultrasonography after isolated limb perfusion. Tumori 2001;87:187–90.

41. Eggimann P, Chiolero R, Chassot PG, et al. Systemic and hemodynamic effects of recombinant tumor necrosis factor alpha in isolation perfusion of the limbs. Chest 1995;107:1074–82.

42. Vrouenraets BC, Klaase JM, Kroon BB, et al. Long-term morbidity after regional isolated perfusion with melphalan for melanoma of the limbs. The influence of acute regional toxic reactions. Arch Surg 1995;130:43–7.

43. Eggermont AM, Schraffordt Koops H, Lienard D, et al. Isolated limb perfusion with high-dose tumor necrosis factor-alpha in combination with interferon-gamma and melphalan for nonresectable extremity soft tissue sarcomas: a multi-center trial. J Clin Oncol 1996;14:2653–65.

44. Bonvalot S, Laplanche A, Lejeune F, et al. Limb salvage with isolated perfusion for soft tissue sarcoma: could less TNF-alpha be better? Ann Oncol 2005;16:1061–8.

45. Rossi CR, Foletto M, Mocellin S, et al. Hyperthermic isolated perfusion with low-dose TNF alpha and doxorubicin in patients with locally advanced soft tissue limb sarcomas. J Chemother 2004;16(Suppl 5):58–61.

46. Di Filippo F, Rossi CR, Vaglini M, et al. Hyperthermic antiblastic perfusion with alpha tumor necrosis factor and doxorubicin for the treatment of soft tissue limb sarcoma in candidates for amputation: results of a phase I study. J Immunother 1999;22:407–14.

47. Rossi CR, Vecchiato A, Foletto M, et al. Phase II study on neoadjuvant hyperthermic-antiblastic perfusion with doxorubicin in patients with intermediate or high grade limb sarcomas. Cancer 1994;73:2140–6.

48. Rouesse JG, Friedman S, Sevin DM, et al. Preoperative induction chemotherapy in the treatment of locally advanced soft tissue sarcomas. Cancer 1987;60: 296–300.

49. Suit HD, Proppe KH, Mankin HJ, et al. Preoperative radiation therapy for sarcoma of soft tissue. Cancer 1981;47:2269–74.

50. Shiu MH, Hilaris BS, Harrison LB, et al. Brachytherapy and function-saving resection of soft tissue sarcoma arising in the limb. Int J Radiat Oncol Biol Phys 1991; 21:1485–92.

51. Lans TE, Grunhagen DJ, de Wilt JG, et al. Isolated limb perfusions with tumor necrosis factor and melphalan for locally recurrent soft tissue sarcoma in previously irradiated limbs. Ann Surg Oncol 2005;12(5):406–11.

52. Olieman AF, van Ginkel RJ, Molenaar WM, et al. Hyperthermic isolated limb perfusion with tumour necrosis factor-alpha and melphalan as palliative limb-saving treatment in patients with locally advanced soft-tissue sarcomas of the extremities with regional or distant metastases. Is it worthwhile? Arch Orthop Trauma Surg 1998;118:70–4.

53. Rossi CR, Mocellin S, Pilati P, et al. Hyperthermic isolated perfusion with low-dose tumor necrosis factor alpha and doxorubicin for the treatment of limb-threatening soft tissue sarcomas. Ann Surg Oncol 2005;12:398–405.

Updates on the Management of Gastrointestinal Stromal Tumors

Zubin M. Bamboat, MD, Ronald P. DeMatteo, MD*

KEYWORDS

- Gastrointestinal stromal tumor • KIT • Tyrosine kinase
- Surgery

EPIDEMIOLOGY

Gastrointestinal stromal tumor (GIST) is the most frequently encountered mesenchymal tumor of the gastrointestinal tract. Although the annual incidence in the United States is reported to be approximately 5000 cases per year,[1] the true incidence is difficult to determine because it was only recently classified as a separate entity from leiomyoma, leiomyosarcoma, and leiomyoblastoma. Because of increased awareness and improved histopathologic detection, the incidence of GIST seems to be increasing.[2] GISTs affect men and women equally, except for pediatric GISTs, which occur predominantly in girls.[3,4] Although GISTs have been reported in all age groups, including newborns, they are uncommon in patients less than 30 years old. Most patients diagnosed with GIST are between 40 and 80 years old, with a median age at diagnosis of 60 years.[5]

The most commonly encountered GIST is the sporadic form. Familial GISTs occur and result from a germline mutation in either the *KIT* or platelet-derived growth factor receptor α (*PDGFRα*) proto-oncogenes.[6,7] GIST can also occur in patients with neurofibromatosis type 1 (NF1)[8] and in young women as part of a syndrome that includes paragangliomas, pulmonary chondromas, and gastric GISTs (ie, the Carney triad).[9]

CLINICAL PRESENTATION AND DIAGNOSIS

GISTs can cause a variety of symptoms ranging from vague abdominal pain to peritonitis as a result of tumor rupture and intraperitoneal bleeding. Other modes of

Funding: This work was supported by NIH Grant CA102613.
Disclosures: Ronald P. DeMatteo is a consultant to and has received honoraria from Novartis.
Department of Surgery, Memorial Sloan-Kettering Cancer Center, 1275 York Avenue, New York, NY 10065, USA
* Corresponding author.
E-mail address: dematter@mskcc.org

Surg Oncol Clin N Am 21 (2012) 301–316
doi:10.1016/j.soc.2011.12.004
1055-3207/12/$ – see front matter © 2012 Published by Elsevier Inc.

presentation include abdominal fullness, early satiety, weakness, and fatigue secondary to anemia from occult gastrointestinal bleeding. Bowel obstruction is rare. Small GISTs (<3 cm) are often detected incidentally on computed tomography (CT) scans, endoscopy, or at the time of laparotomy for other indications.[10] Lesions discovered incidentally and at autopsy have been shown to measure 2.7 cm and 3.4 cm, respectively.[11] Median tumor size at presentation in symptomatic patients is 5 cm.

GISTs can occur anywhere in the gastrointestinal tract from the esophagus to the rectum. The stomach represents the most common site (60%), followed by the small bowel (30%), rectum (~5%), and esophagus (~5%).[5] The clinical course of GIST can range from benign to malignant. Up to 50% of patients present with metastatic disease at the time of diagnosis, with the liver and peritoneum being the 2 most common sites of extraintestinal spread. Occasionally, patients present with primary GISTs of the omentum, mesentery, or pancreas.[12]

Because of the wide range of symptoms and its rarity, the diagnosis of GIST requires a high index of suspicion. The primary mode of diagnosis and assessment of the extent of disease is by contrast-enhanced CT scan of the abdomen and pelvis. Characteristic findings on CT scan include an enhancing, exophytic mass in close association with the stomach or bowel wall. Like other sarcomas, GISTs tend to displace rather than invade adjacent structures. Occasionally, larger GISTs (>10 cm) can show heterogeneity on CT, which usually signifies hemorrhage or occasionally necrosis within the tumor. Magnetic resonance imaging can be useful in cases of rectal GIST. Although positron emission tomography (PET) is not used to diagnose GIST, it can be helpful in assessing the response to tyrosine kinase therapy. PET can also be useful in patients with metastatic disease who are being considered for surgery or those on second-line agents after failure of imatinib, in whom mixed responses may occur. On endoscopic evaluation, GIST appears as a submucosal mass. Although endoscopic or percutaneous biopsy is recommended in cases in which neoadjuvant therapy or metastasis is suspected, the role of routine biopsy of isolated lesions is controversial. Endoscopic-guided fine needle aspiration has been shown to be ~80% sensitive for diagnosing GIST.[13] Because GISTS tend to be soft and friable, biopsy carries the risk of tumor rupture, bleeding, and dissemination.

PATHOLOGIC FINDINGS

There are 3 histologic subtypes of GIST. The spindle cell form is the most common (70%) and consists of uniform, intersecting fascicles with eosinophilic cytoplasm. The epithelioid (20%) and the rare mixed type (10%) forms show more rounded cells with nuclear atypia.[14] Approximately 95% of GISTs stain positive for KIT (CD117) by immunohistochemistry (IHC). Epithelioid GISTs tend to have weaker KIT staining than the spindle cell type. Other commonly expressed markers include CD34 (70%), smooth muscle actin (30%), and desmin (<5%).[14] Although immunophenotype is an important component in the diagnosis of GIST, it is not sufficient. Other malignancies that can stain positive for KIT include metastatic melanoma, angiosarcoma, small cell lung cancer, and Ewing sarcoma.[15] The diagnosis of GIST is based on concordance between the morphology and the IHC. In addition, mutation analysis is sometimes required.

GISTs are believed to arise from the interstitial cells of Cajal as a result of a gain of function mutation in the KIT proto-oncogene. KIT mutations can vary and occur in up to 85% of GISTs.[16] The most common sites of KIT mutation include exon 11 (70%) and exon 9 (10%). Other described regions include exons 13, 14, and 17.[17,18] Recently, ETV1 was shown to be a critical transcription factor in KIT oncogenesis and the development of GISTs.[19] Approximately 10% of patients with GIST instead have a mutation in the *PDGFRα* proto-oncogene.[20] Approximately 5% to 10% of patients do not carry a mutation in either of the proto-oncogenes described earlier and are classed as having wild-type (WT) GISTs. A subset of these patients have a *BRAF* mutation.[21] *DOG1* (a calcium-dependent chloride channel) is also expressed commonly in GIST and can be useful in establishing the diagnosis.[22,23]

RISK STRATIFICATION

Prognosis in GIST is highly variable. The critical determinants of GIST behavior include tumor size, mitotic rate, and location (**Table 1**).[24] Small tumors (<2 cm) with low mitotic rates (<5 per 50 high power fields [HPF]) show benign behavior, whereas larger tumors (>5 cm) with high mitotic rates (>10 per 50 HPF) are associated with malignant behavior and display higher rates of recurrence after surgical resection. Tumors located in the stomach have favorable outcomes relative to small bowel tumors. Of the 3 determinants of behavior mentioned earlier, mitotic rate is considered the most significant.[24] Small tumors with low mitotic rates have still been shown to display malignant behavior.[25]

Gene locus as well as the type of mutation can also affect prognosis. Molecular analysis of the *KIT* proto-oncogene has revealed that tumors with exon 9 mutations or deletions in exon 11 are more aggressive compared with those harboring either a point mutation or insertion in exon 11. Recurrence after surgery is more common in patients with a deletion mutation in exon 11.[24,26,27]

In patients with *PDGFRα* mutations, location is also important. Exon 18 D842V mutations are resistant to imatinib therapy, whereas those in exon 12 are responsive to imatinib. WT GISTs are associated with imatinib resistance and portend an unfavorable prognosis.[28] Insulinlike growth factor receptor 1 (IGFR1) has been shown to be overexpressed in patients with WT GISTs. In vitro suppression of IGFR1 results in apoptosis of imatinib-sensitive and imatinib-resistant WT GIST cells.[29] Trials to

Table 1
Rates of metastases in patients with GISTs of stomach, small bowel, and rectum grouped by tumor size and mitotic rates

	Tumor Parameters		Percentage of Patients with Progressive Disease During Long-term Follow-up and Characterization of Risk for Metastasis			
Group	Size (cm)	Mitotic Rate (per 50 HPF)	Gastric GISTs	Jejunal and Ileal GISTs	Duodenal GISTs	Rectal GISTs
1	≤2	≤5	0, none	0, none	0, none	0, none
2	>2 ≤ 5	≤5	1.9, very low	4.3, low	8.3, low	8.5, low
3a	>5 ≤ 10	≤5	3.6, low	24, moderate	—	—
3b	>10	≤5	12, moderate	52, high	34, high[a]	57, high[a]
4	≤2	>5	0	50	—	54, high
5	>2 ≤ 5	>5	16, moderate	73, high	50, high	52, high
6a	>5 ≤ 10	>5	55, high	85, high	—	—
6b	>10	>5	86, high	90, high	86, high[a]	71, high[a]

[a] Groups 3a and 3b or 6a and 6b are combined in duodenal and rectal GISTs because of the small number of cases.

Data from Miettinen M, Lasota J. Gastrointestinal stromal tumors: pathology and prognosis at different sites. Semin Diagnostic Pathol 2006;23:70.

investigate the efficacy of IGFR1 inhibitors in patients with WT GISTs are under way. More recently, a germline mutation in the succinate dehydrogenase (*SDH*) gene was found in 12% of patients with WT GISTs. Defective cellular respiration as a result of *SDH* mutations in a subset of younger patients with WT GIST is believed to contribute to GIST oncogenesis.[30] Aneuploidy and telomerase expression have both been shown to correlate with worse outcome and the development of metastatic disease.[31–33]

Tumor rupture before or during dissection portends a worse outcome manifested by higher rates of peritoneal recurrence. When examining a specimen, pathologists must consider a slew of prognostic factors that enable them to ultimately categorize GISTs as very low, low, intermediate, or high risk for malignancy.[34] A prognostic nomogram developed at Memorial Sloan-Kettering Cancer Center (MSKCC) that takes into account tumor size, mitotic rate, and location can now be used to assess 2-year and 5-year recurrence-free survival in patients undergoing potentially curative resection of localized primary GIST (**Fig. 1**).[35] Although the nomogram was developed using 127 patients at MSKCC, it has been validated using 2 patient cohorts from other institutions. The fact that inclusion of tyrosine kinase mutation status failed to improve discriminatory ability may reflect only the limited sample size and number of mutation subtypes.

TREATMENT
Primary Resectable Disease

Surgery remains the only chance for cure in patients with localized, primary GIST. The goal is to achieve negative microscopic margins with an intact tumor pseudocapsule. Wide margins have not been shown to improve outcomes.[5] Complete resection can usually be accomplished via wedge resection of the stomach or segmental resection of the bowel. Because GISTs spread hematogenously or by local invasion,

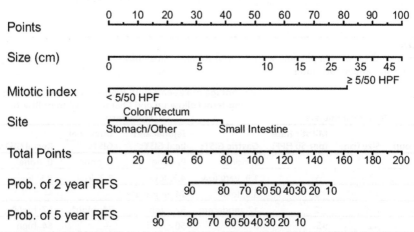

Fig. 1. Nomogram for predicting 2-year and 5-year recurrence-free survival (RFS) in patients with resected localized GIST. An upward vertical line is drawn from the second, third, and fourth rows to the points line. The sum of points generated is marked on the total points line and a vertical line is drawn downward to determine the 2-year and 5-year RFS. (*From* Gold JS, Gonen M, Gutierrez A, et al. Development and validation of a prognostic nomogram for recurrence-free survival after complete surgical resection of localized primary gastrointestinal stromal tumor: a retrospective analysis. Lancet Oncol 2009;10:1048; with permission.)

lymphadenectomy is not routinely required unless adjacent nodes are obviously enlarged. En bloc resection is needed when adjacent organs seem to be involved.

Although there is little disagreement that all tumors larger than 2 cm should be resected, the management of incidentally discovered small GISTs less than 2 cm is controversial. In the absence of high-risk features on endoscopic ultrasonography (EUS) (echogenic foci, ulceration, irregular margins), some have advocated following these lesions with serial imaging or endoscopy. A retrospective analysis looking at the rate of growth of smaller GISTs using EUS found that ~13% with low-risk features on endoscopy progressed to a point at which they were eventually resected.[36] The usefulness of EUS in the management of small GISTs remains unclear. The frequency of imaging is not well defined, and the need for potentially lifelong surveillance makes this option challenging for some patients and physicians. Although endoscopic resection has been suggested by some, the risk of positive margins, perforation, and tumor spillage make this option generally less desirable. Current National Comprehensive Cancer Network (NCCN) guidelines for the management of gastric GISTs less than 2 cm without high-risk features on EUS include surveillance endoscopy every 6 to 12 months.[37]

The role of laparoscopy in the management of patients with GIST continues to expand. The same principles of complete resection with careful intraoperative handling of tumors apply. Laparoscopic resection of localized gastric GISTs has been studied most extensively thus far. A recently published article from MKSCC studied patients with gastric tumors up to 8 cm.[38] Those undergoing laparoscopic resection had equivalent perioperative and oncologic outcomes compared with case-matched controls undergoing open resection. There was no operative mortality, and 30-day morbidity was similar. Oncologic outcomes were also similar, with no positive microscopic margins and 1 recurrence in each group (median follow-up of 34 months). Nishimura and colleagues[39] reported similar results comparing laparoscopic resection with laparotomy in 67 patients with gastric GISTs ranging from 2 to 10 cm.

Adjuvant Therapy

With surgery alone, recurrence rates approached 50% irrespective of negative margins. Conventional adjuvant therapies such as chemotherapy and radiation have not proved effective in GIST. Response rates of 5%[40] have been reported with chemotherapy, and radiation is seldom used because of the difficulty sparing adjacent healthy tissue. Median survival for patients with GIST treated with cytotoxic chemotherapy is approximately 12 months.[41] Moreover, hepatic artery embolization and intraperitoneal chemotherapy have also resulted in discouraging outcomes.[42]

The approval of imatinib mesylate for the treatment of GIST, both adjuvant and therapeutic, has revolutionized the field. As a specific tyrosine kinase inhibitor (TKI), imatinib has shown efficacy in patients with both *KIT* and *PDGFRα* mutations.[43] Imatinib is dosed orally once or twice a day and is generally well tolerated, with rash, diarrhea, and abdominal pain being the most commonly reported side effects.[44]

In a phase II trial led by the American College of Surgeons Oncology Group (ACOSOG), oral imatinib for 12 months after resection in patients with high-risk GISTs was shown to improve recurrence-free survival and increase overall survival compared with historical controls.[45] High risk in this study was defined as a tumor greater than 10 cm, spillage during resection, or more than 5 tumors per patient. In 2009, results from a randomized, placebo-controlled, multicenter phase III trial with 713 patients were reported.[46] Imatinib taken once a day for 1 year after surgery for localized, primary GIST ($\geq$3 cm) was compared with placebo. Recurrence-free survival was significantly higher in the imatinib arm (98%) versus the placebo group (83%) **(Fig. 2)**. Although overall survival was no different, longer follow-up in this patient cohort is needed to definitively determine whether or not adjuvant imatinib can improve overall survival. The cross-over study design may also confound overall survival as an end point. In 2009, the US Food and Drug Administration approved imatinib for use in the adjuvant setting. To define the most effective length of adjuvant imatinib therapy, the results of a recently completed randomized trial comparing 1 year with 3 years of adjuvant imatinib are being finalized. It seems that overall survival is longer with 3 years versus 1 year of adjuvant imatinib.[47] The goal is now to determine which subset of patients with resectable disease truly benefits from adjuvant imatinib. The use of a prognostic nomogram[35] to assess risk of recurrence coupled with mutational analysis may shed some light on this important question.

Primary Unresectable Disease

The role of neoadjuvant imatinib in the setting of locally advanced disease has been investigated. The cytoreductive potential of imatinib in the preoperative setting may enable surgeons to obtain R0 resections with less extensive resections and, therefore, lower morbidity. For example, preoperative therapy for patients with rectal GISTs may increase rates of sphincter-preserving surgery. In addition, tumors located at the gastroesophageal (GE) junction may respond to imatinib such that esophageal resection is avoided. Both rectal and GE junction GISTs have shown shrinkage with neoadjuvant imatinib.[48]

Recent results from a phase II trial led by the Radiation Therapy Oncology Group (RTOG) revealed that imatinib was well tolerated in the neoadjuvant setting.[49] The groups were divided into whether disease was locally advanced and greater than 5 cm (group A) or recurrent/metastatic and greater than 2 cm (group B). Imatinib administered at 600 mg per day for 8 weeks preoperatively was followed by surgery and an additional 2 years of imatinib. This regimen was associated with minimal toxicity and

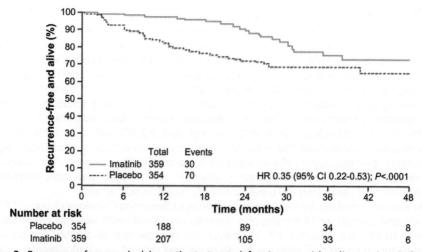

Fig. 2. Recurrence-free survival in patients treated for 1 year with adjuvant imatinib or placebo after resection of localized, primary GIST (≥3 cm). CI, confidence interval; HR, hazard ratio. (*From* DeMatteo RP, Ballman KV, Antonescu CR, et al. Adjuvant imatinib mesylate after resection of localised, primary gastrointestinal stromal tumor: a randomised, double-blind, placebo-controlled trial. Lancet 2009;373(9669):1100; with permission.)

acceptable perioperative complications. Response rates after 8 weeks of preoperative imatinib as determined by response evaluation criteria for solid tumors (RECIST) were similar between groups A and B (4%–7% partial response, 83%–90% stable disease, and 4%–5% progressive disease). The 2-year progression-free survival rates were 83% and 77% in groups A and B, respectively.

Another phase II trial from MD Anderson Cancer Center investigated either 3, 5, or 7 days of neoadjuvant imatinib in 19 patients.[50] All patients received 2 years of postoperative imatinib as well. This regimen was tolerated well and response rates by fluorodeoxyglucose PET were 69%. Median survival for patients treated in this manner was 47 months. There are no published phase III studies investigating the role of neoadjuvant imatinib. The duration of neoadjuvant therapy and patient selection remain to be defined and are at the discretion of the surgeon and medical oncologist. Current NCCN guidelines suggest that, once 2 successive CT scans fail to show any radiographic response for patients on neoadjuvant imatinib, surgical resection should be considered. In general, incomplete resections in patients with advanced disease should be performed only in the setting of palliation of bleeding, pain, or obstruction.

Recurrent and Metastatic Disease

In the preimatinib era, the recurrence rate after resection of primary localized GIST was greater than 50% and the median time to recurrence was 2 years.[5,32] Approximately two-thirds of patients with recurrence have liver metastases and about half have peritoneal disease. A true local recurrence at the site of previous resection is uncommon. Although patients with low metastatic burden were considered for metastasectomy, re-resection alone was almost never curative.

In patients who develop metastases, imatinib is the first line of therapy. Occasionally, patients with symptomatic primary tumors and limited synchronous metastatic disease may be offered surgery before imatinib. The initial report of successfully treating a patient with metastatic GIST using imatinib[51] spurred a series of clinical trials. Up to 80% of patients with metastatic GIST attain a partial or complete response with imatinib.[52] A recent meta-analysis of 2 large, randomized studies[53,54] comparing the efficacy of imatinib 400 mg given either once or twice daily revealed that the higher dose confers a progression-free survival advantage among patients with exon 9 mutations.[55] However, overall survival is unchanged with the higher dose. Because the toxicity of imatinib is dose dependent,[56] current guidelines suggest initiating treatment at a dose of 400 mg per day. Imatinib at 800 mg per day should be considered only as a starting dose for patients with metastatic GIST and a confirmed mutation in exon 9. In patients on 400 mg per day, dose escalation to 800 mg is considered if progression has been documented and toxicity is acceptable. A summary of imatinib trials conducted for metastatic GIST is shown in **Table 2**.

In an effort to improve outcomes in patients with advanced disease, several investigators have looked at combining surgery with imatinib. The rationale for this is based on the fact that a complete pathologic response to imatinib occurs less than 5% of the time. Surgery in patients responding to medical therapy can, therefore, provide the only chance to render them completely free of disease.[57,58] With imatinib, the median survival after surgery for recurrent or metastatic disease has increased from 12 to 15 months to almost 5 years.[53]

Timing of resection and patient selection based on preoperative response to imatinib seem to be critical determinants of outcome. At MSKCC, patients are generally treated with imatinib for about 6 months, after which incremental shrinkage is uncommon. Surgery is then considered.[59] Those who had lesions that were stable or responsive to imatinib had a 2-year progression-free survival of 61% and 2-year

Table 2
Trials of imatinib in metastatic GIST

Trial	Phase	Year	Dose (mg/d) (n)	Follow-Up (Mo)	PR (%)	SD (%)	PD (%)	Notes
EORTC	I	2001, 2002	400, 600, 800, or 1000 (35)	8–12	51	31	8	MTD 800 mg/d
US Multicenter	II	2002, 2004	400 (73)	34	67	16	17	No difference
			800 (74)		66	18	8	
EORTC	III	2003	400 (470)	48	50	32	13	Improved PFS for 800 mg/d
			800 (472)		54	32	9	
Intergroup	III	2003	400 (350)	12	49	22	—	No difference in PFS
			800 (352)		48	22		

Abbreviations: EORTC, European Organisation for Research and Treatment of Cancer; MTD, maximal tolerated dose; PD, progressive disease; PFS, progression-free survival; PR, partial response; SD, stable disease.

overall survival of 100% after surgical resection. In contrast, patients with focal resistance or multiple lesions that were resistant to imatinib did considerably worse, with a 2-year overall survival of only 36%. A similar study in 67 patients by Raut and colleagues[60] confirmed that debulking surgery has little to offer patients with progressive metastatic disease, but might prolong survival in those who are either responsive to imatinib or have limited radiographic progression. Twelve-month progression-free survival was 80%, 33%, and 0% for patients with stable disease, limited progression, and widespread progression, respectively. A study by Gronchi and colleagues,[61] confirmed that surgery may be of value to a select subset of patients who develop responsive or stable disease while on TKI therapy. The recommended duration of therapy for patients who are responding to imatinib is not well established. Most experts consider surgery after 6 to 12 months of medical therapy, given the estimated time for development of secondary mutations is 2 years.[62] ACOSOG and the European Organisation for Research and Treatment of Cancer have unsuccessfully attempted to assess the efficacy of surgery for locally advanced or metastatic GIST in combination with continued TKI therapy.

Other treatment options for patients with advanced disease include radiofrequency ablation (RFA), hepatic artery embolization, and liver transplantation. RFA is typically reserved for patients with unresectable liver disease. Select patients with multiple liver metastases can undergo combined resection with RFA. The use of hepatic artery embolization is reserved for patients with a significant hepatic metastatic burden who have failed multiple TKIs.[63,64] There have been only a few case reports of patients undergoing liver transplantation for metastatic GIST.[65] The role of transplantation for metastatic disease remains uncertain.

Treatment of Imatinib-resistant Disease

Primary resistance to imatinib is defined as the development of radiographic progression during the first 6 months of treatment. Size is not the sole criterion by which radiographic response is measured. GISTs can develop areas of necrosis and maintain the same size and appearance on CT scan. In the absence of progressive disease, traditional RECIST criteria may be of limited usefulness in assessing response to TKI therapy.[66] The best available option at this time may be to use modified RECIST criteria, in which tumor density in addition to size is measured by CT scan.[67] Determination of responsive disease may sometimes require functional assessment of tumors using PET.

The presence and location of mutations in KIT and PDGFRα can provide insight into the mechanism of resistance. WT GISTs, or those that contain mutations in exon 9 of KIT or a D842V mutation in PDGFRα, are likely to show primary resistance. Secondary resistance occurs later in the course of imatinib therapy (>6 months), most often as the result of a second mutation in the kinase domain of KIT or PDGFRα.[68–70] Most GISTs that develop secondary imatinib resistance have a primary mutation in KIT exon 11 and then develop an exon 13, 14, or 17 KIT mutation.

The second-line agent for patients with imatinib-resistant disease is sunitinib.[71] Sunitinib targets KIT and PDGFRα as well as the vascular endothelial cell growth factor receptor, fms-like tyrosine kinase 3 receptor, and the RET receptor. In patients with advanced disease resistant to imatinib, a randomized trial has shown that sunitinib is a safe and effective second-line agent.[72] Patients randomized to the sunitinib arm had a median time to progression of 7 months compared with 1.5 months for the placebo arm. Tolerability was acceptable, with the most common side effects being fatigue, diarrhea, skin discoloration, and nausea. Raut and colleagues[73] investigated the potential benefit of surgery in patients with advanced disease resistant to imatinib.

Fifty patients underwent surgery after a median time of 6.7 months on sunitinib therapy. Median progression-free survival after surgery was 6 months and median overall survival was 16 months. Response to sunitinib at the time of surgery did not correlate with postoperative progression-free survival. Incomplete resections and complication rates were relatively high at 50%. The potential benefits of surgery for patients with advanced disease on second-line TKI therapy needs to be carefully weighed against the risks on an individual basis.

Options for patients with disease refractory to imatinib and sunitinib are limited. Although several third-line agents such as sorafenib, nilotinib, dasatinib, and, most recently, vatalanib[74] have been used in some patients, there is no clear optimal third-line agent. Partial responses and stable disease in patients treated with sorafenib have been reported.[75,76] A phase III trial from the Cancer and Leukemia Group B is under way comparing sorafenib with nilotinib in patients with GIST resistant to imatinib and sunitinib.

PEDIATRIC GIST

Pediatric GISTs are different from those occurring in the adult population. In contrast to adult GISTs, pediatric GISTs are more indolent, display higher rates of recurrence, and are more common in girls.[37] Mutations in *KIT* and *PDGFRα* are uncommon in the pediatric population and most patients are WT for both proto-oncogenes.[4] As a result, response rates to imatinib in this population are lower compared with adults. A recent study reported that *SDH* might play an important role in the oncogenesis of WT GISTs in younger patients.[30] Surgery remains the only chance for cure in children. A complete mutational analysis, including *SDH,* and referral to a specialty center or the National Institutes of Health pediatric GIST clinic is recommended for pediatric patients diagnosed with GIST.

FAMILIAL GIST

Familial GISTs are characterized by germline mutations in either *KIT* or *PDGFRα*. Patients often present with associated abnormalities such as skin hyperpigmentation and a history of irritable bowel syndrome. Tumors tend to be multifocal, occur more commonly in the small bowel, and frequently have a low mitotic rate. Unlike sporadic GISTs, the type of mutation does not seem to affect the clinical course.[77] Response to TKIs is uncertain.

FUTURE STRATEGIES

Novel approaches aimed at enhancing response rates and reducing recurrence include combining TKI therapy with radiotherapy.[78] Phase II trials are under way using sunitinib with radiation in patients with progressive disease on imatinib. Although investigational third-line TKIs such as nilotinib, dasatinib, sorafenib, and vatalanib have shown some promise in patients with disease refractory to imatinib and sunitinib, additional targets of the oncogenic pathway are needed. Phase III trials looking at the efficacy of other pathways such as mammalian target of rapamycin and heat shock proteins, are currently being performed. With the recent discovery that *BRAF* mutations exist in a subset of patients with WT GISTs,[21] the use of BRAF inhibitors is also being investigated.

Another innovative strategy that may show promise involves combining TKI therapy with immunomodulation. In a murine model, we recently found that part of the effects of imatinib on GIST is mediated by the immune system. This mechanism depended on

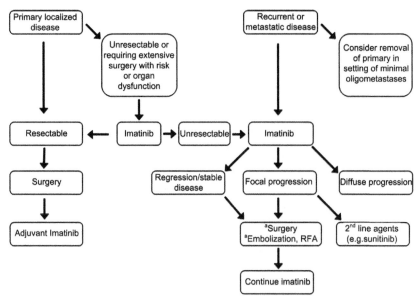

Fig. 3. Algorithm for the management of GIST. [a]If all gross disease or all imatinib-resistant disease is treatable.

imatinib lowering tumor production of indoleamine 2,3-dioxygenase, an immunosuppressive protein that blocks T-cell function.[79] The addition of ipilimumab (Yervoy) to TKI therapy may further enable tumor-specific T cells to kill GIST.

SUMMARY

The goals in treating patients with GIST are to maximize the chance of cure, minimize recurrence, limit the metastatic burden, and maintain a reasonable quality of life. A multidisciplinary approach to patients with GISTs is necessary to optimize the timing of medical and surgical therapy. An evidence-based treatment algorithm is outlined in **Fig. 3**.

REFERENCES

1. Demetri GD, Baker LH, Benjamin RS, et al. Soft tissue sarcoma. J Natl Compr Canc Netw 2007;5(4):364–99.
2. Steigen SE, Eide TJ. Trends in incidence and survival of mesenchymal neoplasm of the digestive tract within a defined population of northern Norway. APMIS 2006; 114(3):192–200.
3. Tran T, Davila JA, El-Serag HB. The epidemiology of malignant gastrointestinal stromal tumors: an analysis of 1,458 cases from 1992 to 2000. Am J Gastroenterol 2005;100(1):162–8.
4. Prakash S, Sarran L, Socci N, et al. Gastrointestinal stromal tumors in children and young adults: a clinicopathologic, molecular, and genomic study of 15 cases and review of the literature. J Pediatr Hematol Oncol 2005;27(4):179–87.
5. DeMatteo RP, Lewis JJ, Leung D, et al. Two hundred gastrointestinal stromal tumors: recurrence patterns and prognostic factors for survival. Ann Surg 2000;231(1):51–8.

6. Nishida T, Hirota S, Taniguchi M, et al. Familial gastrointestinal stromal tumours with germline mutation of the KIT gene. Nat Genet 1998;19(4):323–4.

7. Chompret A, Kannengiesser C, Barrois M, et al. PDGFRA germline mutation in a family with multiple cases of gastrointestinal stromal tumor. Gastroenterology 2004;126(1):318–21.

8. Takazawa Y, Sakurai S, Sakuma Y, et al. Gastrointestinal stromal tumors of neurofibromatosis type I (von Recklinghausen's disease). Am J Surg Pathol 2005;29(6): 755–63.

9. Carney JA. The triad of gastric epithelioid leiomyosarcoma, functioning extraadrenal paraganglioma, and pulmonary chondroma. Cancer 1979;43(1):374–82.

10. van der Zwan SM, DeMatteo RP. Gastrointestinal stromal tumor: 5 years later. Cancer 2005;104(9):1781–8.

11. Nilsson B, Bumming P, Meis-Kindblom JM, et al. Gastrointestinal stromal tumors: the incidence, prevalence, clinical course, and prognostication in the preimatinib mesylate era–a population-based study in western Sweden. Cancer 2005;103(4): 821–9.

12. Graadt van Roggen JF, van Velthuysen ML, Hogendoorn PC. The histopathological differential diagnosis of gastrointestinal stromal tumours. J Clin Pathol 2001; 54(2):96–102.

13. Sepe PS, Moparty B, Pitman MB, et al. EUS-guided FNA for the diagnosis of GI stromal cell tumors: sensitivity and cytologic yield. Gastrointest Endosc 2009; 70(2):254–61.

14. Fletcher CD, Berman JJ, Corless C, et al. Diagnosis of gastrointestinal stromal tumors: a consensus approach. Hum Pathol 2002;33(5):459–65.

15. Miettinen M, Lasota J. KIT (CD117): a review on expression in normal and neoplastic tissues, and mutations and their clinicopathologic correlation. Appl Immunohistochem Mol Morphol 2005;13(3):205–20.

16. Rubin BP, Singer S, Tsao C, et al. KIT activation is a ubiquitous feature of gastrointestinal stromal tumors. Cancer Res 2001;61(22):8118–21.

17. Antonescu CR, Sommer G, Sarran L, et al. Association of KIT exon 9 mutations with nongastric primary site and aggressive behavior: KIT mutation analysis and clinical correlates of 120 gastrointestinal stromal tumors. Clin Cancer Res 2003;9(9):3329–37.

18. Lux ML, Rubin BP, Biase TL, et al. KIT extracellular and kinase domain mutations in gastrointestinal stromal tumors. Am J Pathol 2000;156(3):791–5.

19. Chi P, Chen Y, Zhang L, et al. ETV1 is a lineage survival factor that cooperates with KIT in gastrointestinal stromal tumours. Nature 2010;467(7317):849–53.

20. Heinrich MC, Corless CL, Duensing A, et al. PDGFRA activating mutations in gastrointestinal stromal tumors. Science 2003;299(5607):708–10.

21. Agaram NP, Wong GC, Guo T, et al. Novel V600E BRAF mutations in imatinib-naive and imatinib-resistant gastrointestinal stromal tumors. Genes Chromosomes Cancer 2008;47(10):853–9.

22. Espinosa I, Lee CH, Kim MK, et al. A novel monoclonal antibody against DOG1 is a sensitive and specific marker for gastrointestinal stromal tumors. Am J Surg Pathol 2008;32(2):210–8.

23. West RB, Corless CL, Chen X, et al. The novel marker, DOG1, is expressed ubiquitously in gastrointestinal stromal tumors irrespective of KIT or PDGFRA mutation status. Am J Pathol 2004;165(1):107–13.

24. Dematteo RP, Gold JS, Saran L, et al. Tumor mitotic rate, size, and location independently predict recurrence after resection of primary gastrointestinal stromal tumor (GIST). Cancer 2008;112(3):608–15.

25. Franquemont DW. Differentiation and risk assessment of gastrointestinal stromal tumors. Am J Clin Pathol 1995;103(1):41–7.
26. Martin J, Poveda A, Llombart-Bosch A, et al. Deletions affecting codons 557-558 of the c-KIT gene indicate a poor prognosis in patients with completely resected gastrointestinal stromal tumors: a study by the Spanish Group for Sarcoma Research (GEIS). J Clin Oncol 2005;23(25):6190–8.
27. Debiec-Rychter M, Sciot R, Le Cesne A, et al. KIT mutations and dose selection for imatinib in patients with advanced gastrointestinal stromal tumours. Eur J Cancer 2006;42(8):1093–103.
28. Debiec-Rychter M, Wasag B, Stul M, et al. Gastrointestinal stromal tumours (GISTs) negative for KIT (CD117 antigen) immunoreactivity. J Pathol 2004; 202(4):430–8.
29. Tarn C, Rink L, Merkel E, et al. Insulin-like growth factor 1 receptor is a potential therapeutic target for gastrointestinal stromal tumors. Proc Natl Acad Sci U S A 2008;105(24):8387–92.
30. Janeway KA, Kim SY, Lodish M, et al. Defects in succinate dehydrogenase in gastrointestinal stromal tumors lacking KIT and PDGFRA mutations. Proc Natl Acad Sci U S A 2011;108(1):314–8.
31. Rudolph P, Gloeckner K, Parwaresch R, et al. Immunophenotype, proliferation, DNA ploidy, and biological behavior of gastrointestinal stromal tumors: a multivariate clinicopathologic study. Hum Pathol 1998;29(8):791–800.
32. Ng EH, Pollock RE, Munsell MF, et al. Prognostic factors influencing survival in gastrointestinal leiomyosarcomas. Implications for surgical management and staging. Ann Surg 1992;215(1):68–77.
33. Gunther T, Schneider-Stock R, Hackel C, et al. Telomerase activity and expression of hTRT and hTR in gastrointestinal stromal tumors in comparison with extra-gastrointestinal sarcomas. Clin Cancer Res 2000;6(5):1811–8.
34. Miettinen M, Lasota J. Gastrointestinal stromal tumors: pathology and prognosis at different sites. Semin Diagn Pathol 2006;23(2):70–83.
35. Gold JS, Gonen M, Gutierrez A, et al. Development and validation of a prognostic nomogram for recurrence-free survival after complete surgical resection of localised primary gastrointestinal stromal tumour: a retrospective analysis. Lancet Oncol 2009;10(11):1045–52.
36. Lok KH, Lai L, Yiu HL, et al. Endosonographic surveillance of small gastrointestinal tumors originating from muscularis propria. J Gastrointestin Liver Dis 2009;18(2):177–80.
37. Demetri GD, von Mehren M, Antonescu CR, et al. NCCN Task Force report: update on the management of patients with gastrointestinal stromal tumors. J Natl Compr Canc Netw 2010;8(Suppl 2):S1–41 [quiz: S2–4].
38. Karakousis GC, Singer S, Zheng J, et al. Laparoscopic versus open gastric resections for primary gastrointestinal stromal tumors (GISTs): a size-matched comparison. Ann Surg Oncol 2011;18(6):1599–605.
39. Nishimura J, Nakajima K, Omori T, et al. Surgical strategy for gastric gastrointestinal stromal tumors: laparoscopic vs. open resection. Surg Endosc 2007;21(6): 875–8.
40. Dematteo RP, Heinrich MC, El-Rifai WM, et al. Clinical management of gastrointestinal stromal tumors: before and after STI-571. Hum Pathol 2002;33(5):466–77.
41. Edmonson JH, Marks RS, Buckner JC, et al. Contrast of response to dacarbazine, mitomycin, doxorubicin, and cisplatin (DMAP) plus GM-CSF between patients with advanced malignant gastrointestinal stromal tumors and patients with other advanced leiomyosarcomas. Cancer Invest 2002;20(5–6):605–12.

42. D'Amato G, Steinert DM, McAuliffe JC, et al. Update on the biology and therapy of gastrointestinal stromal tumors. Cancer Control 2005;12(1):44–56.
43. Savage DG, Antman KH. Imatinib mesylate–a new oral targeted therapy. N Engl J Med 2002;346(9):683–93.
44. Demetri GD, von Mehren M, Blanke CD, et al. Efficacy and safety of imatinib mesylate in advanced gastrointestinal stromal tumors. N Engl J Med 2002;347(7):472–80.
45. Dematteo RP, Owzar K, Antonescu CR, et al. Efficacy of adjuvant imatinib mesylate following complete resection of localized, primary gastrointestinal stromal tumor (GIST) at high risk of recurrence: the U.S. Intergroup phase II trial ACOSOG Z9000. In: American Society of Clinical Oncology 2008 Gastrointestinal Cancers Symposium. Orlando (FL); 2008. p. A8.
46. Dematteo RP, Ballman KV, Antonescu CR, et al. Adjuvant imatinib mesylate after resection of localised, primary gastrointestinal stromal tumour: a randomised, double-blind, placebo-controlled trial. Lancet 2009;373(9669):1097–104.
47. Joensuu H. Twelve versus 36 months of adjuvant imatinib (IM) as treatment of operable GIST with a high risk of recurrence: final results of a randomized trial. J Clin Oncol 2011;29(Suppl; abstract LBA1).
48. Hohenberger P, Oladeji O, Licht T, et al. Neoadjuvant imatinib and organ preservation in locally advanced gastrointestinal stromal tumors (GIST) [abstract: 10550]. J Clin Oncol 2009;27(Suppl 1).
49. Eisenberg BL, Harris J, Blanke CD, et al. Phase II trial of neoadjuvant/adjuvant imatinib mesylate (IM) for advanced primary and metastatic/recurrent operable gastrointestinal stromal tumor (GIST): early results of RTOG 0132/ACRIN 6665. J Surg Oncol 2009;99(1):42–7.
50. McAuliffe JC, Hunt KK, Lazar AJ, et al. A randomized, phase II study of preoperative plus postoperative imatinib in GIST: evidence of rapid radiographic response and temporal induction of tumor cell apoptosis. Ann Surg Oncol 2009;16(4):910–9.
51. Joensuu H, Roberts PJ, Sarlomo-Rikala M, et al. Effect of the tyrosine kinase inhibitor STI571 in a patient with a metastatic gastrointestinal stromal tumor. N Engl J Med 2001;344(14):1052–6.
52. Katz SC, DeMatteo RP. Gastrointestinal stromal tumors and leiomyosarcomas. J Surg Oncol 2008;97(4):350–9.
53. Verweij J, Casali PG, Zalcberg J, et al. Progression-free survival in gastrointestinal stromal tumours with high-dose imatinib: randomised trial. Lancet 2004; 364(9440):1127–34.
54. Blanke CD, Rankin C, Demetri GD, et al. Phase III randomized, intergroup trial assessing imatinib mesylate at two dose levels in patients with unresectable or metastatic gastrointestinal stromal tumors expressing the kit receptor tyrosine kinase: S0033. J Clin Oncol 2008;26(4):626–32.
55. (MetaGIST) GSTM-AG. Comparison of two doses of imatinib for the treatment of unresectable or metastatic gastrointestinal stromal tumors: a meta-analysis of 1,640 patients. J Clin Oncol 2010;28(7):1247–53.
56. Van Glabbeke M, Verweij J, Casali PG, et al. Predicting toxicities for patients with advanced gastrointestinal stromal tumours treated with imatinib: a study of the European Organisation for Research and Treatment of Cancer, the Italian Sarcoma Group, and the Australasian Gastro-Intestinal Trials Group (EORTC-ISG-AGITG). Eur J Cancer 2006;42(14):2277–85.
57. Bumming P, Andersson J, Meis-Kindblom JM, et al. Neoadjuvant, adjuvant and palliative treatment of gastrointestinal stromal tumours (GIST) with imatinib: a centre-based study of 17 patients. Br J Cancer 2003;89(3):460–4.

58. Bauer S, Hartmann JT, de Wit M, et al. Resection of residual disease in patients with metastatic gastrointestinal stromal tumors responding to treatment with imatinib. Int J Cancer 2005;117(2):316–25.

59. DeMatteo RP, Maki RG, Singer S, et al. Results of tyrosine kinase inhibitor therapy followed by surgical resection for metastatic gastrointestinal stromal tumor. Ann Surg 2007;245(3):347–52.

60. Raut CP, Posner M, Desai J, et al. Surgical management of advanced gastrointestinal stromal tumors after treatment with targeted systemic therapy using kinase inhibitors. J Clin Oncol 2006;24(15):2325–31.

61. Gronchi A, Fiore M, Miselli F, et al. Surgery of residual disease following molecular-targeted therapy with imatinib mesylate in advanced/metastatic GIST. Ann Surg 2007;245(3):341–6.

62. Blanke CD, Demetri GD, von Mehren M, et al. Long-term results from a randomized phase II trial of standard- versus higher-dose imatinib mesylate for patients with unresectable or metastatic gastrointestinal stromal tumors expressing KIT. J Clin Oncol 2008;26(4):620–5.

63. Kobayashi K, Szklaruk J, Trent JC, et al. Hepatic arterial embolization and chemoembolization for imatinib-resistant gastrointestinal stromal tumors. Am J Clin Oncol 2009;32(6):574–81.

64. Kobayashi K, Gupta S, Trent JC, et al. Hepatic artery chemoembolization for 110 gastrointestinal stromal tumors: response, survival, and prognostic factors. Cancer 2006;107(12):2833–41.

65. Serralta AS, Sanjuan FR, Moya AH, et al. Combined liver transplantation plus imatinib for unresectable metastases of gastrointestinal stromal tumours. Eur J Gastroenterol Hepatol 2004;16(11):1237–9.

66. Benjamin RS, Choi H, Macapinlac HA, et al. We should desist using RECIST, at least in GIST. J Clin Oncol 2007;25(13):1760–4.

67. Choi H, Charnsangavej C, Faria SC, et al. Correlation of computed tomography and positron emission tomography in patients with metastatic gastrointestinal stromal tumor treated at a single institution with imatinib mesylate: proposal of new computed tomography response criteria. J Clin Oncol 2007;25(13):1753–9.

68. Chen LL, Trent JC, Wu EF, et al. A missense mutation in KIT kinase domain 1 correlates with imatinib resistance in gastrointestinal stromal tumors. Cancer Res 2004;64(17):5913–9.

69. Debiec-Rychter M, Cools J, Dumez H, et al. Mechanisms of resistance to imatinib mesylate in gastrointestinal stromal tumors and activity of the PKC412 inhibitor against imatinib-resistant mutants. Gastroenterology 2005; 128(2):270–9.

70. Antonescu CR, Besmer P, Guo T, et al. Acquired resistance to imatinib in gastrointestinal stromal tumor occurs through secondary gene mutation. Clin Cancer Res 2005;11(11):4182–90.

71. Prenen H, Cools J, Mentens N, et al. Efficacy of the kinase inhibitor SU11248 against gastrointestinal stromal tumor mutants refractory to imatinib mesylate. Clin Cancer Res 2006;12(8):2622–7.

72. Demetri GD, van Oosterom AT, Garrett CR, et al. Efficacy and safety of sunitinib in patients with advanced gastrointestinal stromal tumour after failure of imatinib: a randomised controlled trial. Lancet 2006;368(9544):1329–38.

73. Raut CP, Wang Q, Manola J, et al. Cytoreductive surgery in patients with metastatic gastrointestinal stromal tumor treated with sunitinib malate. Ann Surg Oncol 2010;17(2):407–15.

74. Joensuu H, De Braud F, Grignagni G, et al. Vatalanib for metastatic gastrointestinal stromal tumour (GIST) resistant to imatinib: final results of a phase II study. Br J Cancer 2011;104(11):1686–90.
75. Wiebe L, Kasza KE, Maki RG, et al. Activity of sorafenib (SOR) in patients (pts) with imatinib (IM) and sunitinib (SU)-resistant (RES) gastrointestinal stromal tumors (GIST): a phase II trial of the University of Chicago Phase II Consortium [abstract 10502]. J Clin Oncol 2008;26(Suppl 1).
76. Reichardt P, Montemurro M, Gelderblom H, et al. Sorafenib fourth-line treatment in imatinib-, sunitinib-, and nilotinib-resistant metastatic GIST: a retrospective analysis [abstract: 10564]. J Clin Oncol 2009;27(Suppl 1).
77. Antonescu CR. Gastrointestinal stromal tumor (GIST) pathogenesis, familial GIST, and animal models. Semin Diagn Pathol 2006;23(2):63–9.
78. Kao J, Packer S, Vu HL, et al. Phase 1 study of concurrent sunitinib and image-guided radiotherapy followed by maintenance sunitinib for patients with oligometastases: acute toxicity and preliminary response. Cancer 2009;115(15):3571–80.
79. Balachandran VP, Cavnar M, Zeng S, et al. Imatinib mesylate potentiates anti-tumor T cell responses in gastrointestinal stromal tumor through the inhibition of indoleamine 2,3-dioxygenase. Nat Med 2011;17(9):1094–100.

Improving Outcomes for Retroperitoneal Sarcomas: A Work in Progress

Carol J. Swallow, MD, PhD, FRCS[a,b,]*, Charles N. Catton, MD, FRCP[c,d]

KEYWORDS

- Retroperitoneal sarcoma • Long-term outcomes
- Soft tissue sarcoma • Liposarcoma

Retroperitoneal sarcoma (RPS) represents 10% to 15% of all soft tissue sarcoma (STS), with a stable annual incidence of approximately 2.7 cases per 1 million persons in the United States.[1] A similar incidence has been reported for the population of southern Sweden.[2] The disease has no apparent geographic variation in incidence and no predisposition by gender or race. In patients with hereditary or sporadic genetic conditions that predispose to STS, the proportion of these tumors that arise in the retroperitoneum is not appreciably different from that in the general population. However, the distribution of histologic subtypes in RPS differs from that of STS arising at other anatomic sites. Approximately 50% of RPSs are liposarcoma. The second most frequent histology is leiomyosarcoma; a small proportion will arise from the smooth muscle of the inferior vena cava (IVC). Ongoing debate surrounds whether other histologic subtypes exist (eg, malignant fibrous histiocytoma [MFH], pleomorphic sarcoma); some authors suggest that many of these are, in fact, dedifferentiated liposarcoma.

Currently, no consensus exists in the literature regarding the need for a pretreatment percutaneous biopsy of a suspected RPS. Given that the differential diagnosis is actually fairly broad (eg, lymphoma, testicular/germ cell tumors, benign or malignant adrenal/renal tumors, benign peripheral nerve sheath tumors, ganglioneuroma,

[a] Department of Surgery, University of Toronto, Mount Sinai Hospital, 600 University Avenue, Suite 1225, Toronto, Ontario, Canada M5G 1X5
[b] Department of Surgical Oncology, Princess Margaret Hospital, 610 University Avenue, 3rd Floor, Toronto, Canada
[c] Department of Radiation Oncology, University of Toronto, Toronto, Canada
[d] Radiation Medicine Program, Princess Margaret Hospital, 610 University Avenue, 5th Floor, Toronto, Canada
* Corresponding author. Department of Surgery, University of Toronto, Mount Sinai Hospital, 600 University Avenue, Suite 1225, Toronto, Ontario, Canada M5G 1X5.
E-mail address: cswallow@mtsinai.on.ca

Surg Oncol Clin N Am 21 (2012) 317–331
doi:10.1016/j.soc.2012.01.002
1055-3207/12/$ – see front matter © 2012 Elsevier Inc. All rights reserved.

lymphangioma, retroperitoneal fibrosis, metastatic carcinoma) with widely differing treatments, the benefits of securing a histologic diagnosis before formulating a treatment plan outweigh the theoretical risk of tumor seeding along the biopsy track. Furthermore, if neoadjuvant treatment is being contemplated, confirming the RPS diagnosis is important. Fine needle aspiration biopsy is of little use because a pathologic diagnosis commonly relies on tissue architecture; therefore, core biopsy is strongly preferred. With modern techniques, including withdrawal of the core needle and specimen into the hub of the biopsy gun, and sophisticated image guidance, the potential for tumor contamination of surrounding tissues is minimized. In contrast, open surgical biopsy of a suspected RPS is much more likely than a percutaneous biopsy to expose virgin tissue planes to tumor and miss viable tumor material, and requires a sizable incision with attendant risks. Therefore, open biopsy should be used only if repeated percutaneous biopsies have failed and the management would change based on a definitive RPS diagnosis.

Surgical resection remains the cornerstone of RPS treatment. In the United States from 1973 to 2001, the resection rate has increased; it is currently approximately 80%. Several reports indicate that resectability may be optimized by referral to specialized centers.[3] However, an attempt at resection may not be appropriate in all cases, because the presence of distant metastatic disease or poor patient performance status can portend abbreviated survival regardless of treatment. Resection as a sole therapeutic modality has resulted in 5-year local recurrence rates of 50% to 70% and 5-year overall survival rates of 40% to 50%.[4] Local recurrence and death from sarcoma continue at a significant rate beyond 10 years, and even up to 20 years after resection.[5,6]

Given the failure of surgery alone to control most RPS, considerable interest has been shown in adjuvant therapies. Except for particularly chemosensitive histologies, such as extraosseous Ewing's, chemotherapy in general has not been systematically used. Because of the success of radiation therapy (RT) at reducing local recurrence of extremity STS, its potential benefit in RPS (in which margins are typically compromised) has been explored. Before 2001, RT was used in approximately 25% of patients with RPS undergoing resection (postoperatively in 75% of cases).[1,6] Postoperative RT is limited by toxicity and does not seem to prevent recurrence; it has been largely abandoned at many experienced centers. The role of preoperative RT remains unclear, as discussed later in this article.

RPS CLINICAL OUTCOME MEASURES
Local Recurrence

RPS has a marked propensity to recur locoregionally within the abdominal cavity, as opposed to at distant sites from hematogenous dissemination. In particular, patients with liposarcoma rarely develop distant metastases.[7] The mechanism of death from recurrent RPS is most frequently related to progression of locoregional recurrence or complications of its treatment. Thus, RPS local progression-free survival closely mimics overall cancer-specific survival.[8] Although complete gross resection of a locoregional recurrence is often technically feasible and some patients undergo multiple resections, these are highly selected cases. Therefore, reports on the results of resection of recurrent disease are prone to significant selection bias. Patients who experience recurrence with an aggressive, technically unresectable tumor are usually not included in surgical series. Those who experience recurrence with more indolent, resectable disease are noted to have a surprisingly favorable survival, probably reflecting tumor biology as much as a beneficial treatment effect.

Baseline postresection imaging, typically a CT scan with both oral and intravenous contrast, is critical to act as a comparator for future surveillance studies. Radiologic evidence of RPS recurrence often predates the development of symptoms. For low-grade tumors, this interval can sometimes be measured in years. Survival after resection of an asymptomatic local recurrence might be superior to resection of a symptomatic recurrence, but this may simply reflect lead-time bias. Another issue related to assessing RPS treatment outcomes is the confirmation of a local recurrence; sometimes it requires serial imaging to definitively document progressive disease. Whether the date of recurrence should be reported as that of the first suspicious scan or the ensuing confirmatory scans is unclear. In addition, the interval between scans during long-term follow-up can often be 1 to 2 years, further confounding this outcome measure.

The risk for local recurrence of RPS occurs at a significant rate even after 5 years following curative intent surgery.[9] For LPS, local recurrence rates 5 years after complete gross resection are approximately 50% for well-differentiated and 80% for dedifferentiated tumors.[10,11] In studies that include longer follow-up, local recurrence risk does not plateau at 5 years, but instead continues at a near-linear pace. Therefore, the follow-up of patients with RPS assumes a lifelong aspect, highlighting the importance of institutional commitment to the follow-up of these patients and also the difficulties of designing clinical trials that can be concluded within a reasonable time-frame.

Overall Survival

RPS is distinct from STS at other sites in that cancer-specific survival continues to decline significantly beyond 5 and even 10 years after resection.[5,8,12,13] Most older published series (single-institution series collected over 20 to 30 years using surgery alone) note 5-year overall survival rates of 50%. More recent population-based estimates are similar to these older series, also showing 5-year overall survival rates of approximately 50%.[12,13] In studies that include longer follow-up, 10-year actuarial disease-related survival decreases to 20% to 30%, again highlighting the importance of extended follow-up in assessing RPS treatment outcomes.

PROGNOSTIC VARIABLES FOR RPS OUTCOME

The failing of the American Joint Committee on Cancer (AJCC) STS staging system as applied to RPS outcomes has been emphasized by several authors.[3,13] Very few of these tumors are smaller than 5 cm, with the median maximal dimension in most series being 25 to 30 cm. By definition, all RPS are deep. Distant metastases are uncommon at diagnosis but do predict poor survival when present. The element of the AJCC system most valuable in predicting outcome in RPS is grade. Grade and resection status are the two prognostic factors recognized as useful for comparing outcomes between series and in counseling individual patients. Although resection status and grade are interrelated, with high-grade tumors less likely to be completely resected, the two variables are still independent predictors of prognosis in most larger series.[12]

Grade

Grade is consistently found to be an important prognostic factor in most RPS series, including an analysis of 1535 patients from the Surveillance, Epidemiology, and End Results (SEER) database.[5,6,10,14–18] Using the French three-tier grading system, Bonvalot and colleagues[9] showed that grade was the most significant independent predictor of abdominal recurrence-free and overall survival in 364 patients with resected primary RPS. An analysis of 261 cases of primary RPS from merged tumor registries from more than 150 United States centers yielded similar results for high versus low grade.[19] Grobmyer and colleagues[20] analyzed 78 cases of recurrent RPS and also found that high-grade tumor was an independent predictor of worse overall survival.

Resection (R) status

R0 resection (histologically confirmed circumferentially negative margins) is the universally upheld goal of RPS surgery. In practice, its achievement is challenging and, some would argue, illusory. With large tumors, it is not technically feasible to pathologically examine all margins of resection. Areas of concern identified by the surgeon or pathologist should be specifically assessed. Pathologic analysis may reveal tumor within a particular distance of the margin of resection, such as within 0.1 mm; this resection would then be labeled R1. Variations in the sampling intervals of the circumference of the tumor and the strictness with which measurements are made likely account for the wide variations in the R0 versus R1 rates reported in the literature (**Table 1**).

Despite the noted limitations, R status has been identified as a significant predictor of local recurrence and overall survival for resected RPS. Singer and colleagues[10] were among the first to emphasize that R status, which is not a component of AJCC/International Union Against Cancer (UICC) staging, trumps every other staging element in patients with no obvious distant metastatic disease. Patients who have undergone an R2 resection have inferior overall survival compared with R0 or R1 resection. In some reports, R2 resection rates are markedly lower at specialized centers versus community hospitals. Although this may reflect a more aggressive surgical approach, it may also suggest better patient selection based on review of preoperative imaging. Because the goal of surgery should be complete gross tumor resection, the potential benefits of incomplete resection remain controversial. Some series have shown that overall survival is longer in patients who have undergone R2 resection than in those who did not undergo surgical exploration. In this regard, a significant source of bias and also heterogeneity between series is in patient selection. For example, in most series in which patients had an R2 resection, that was not the intent of the planned surgery. Rather, they were taken to the operating room with the plan of performing a total gross resection. Therefore, this group would be different a priori from patients in whom the imaging suggested an inability to perform a complete resection, thus precluding surgical exploration.

Primary Versus Recurrent Tumor

For the most part, large population-based analyses and multi-institutional series have focused on primary RPS. Most available information on patients with recurrent RPS comes from small retrospective surgical series. These series typically are composed of patients who underwent resection or were at least subjected to laparotomy with the intent of a curative resection. There is almost certainly a major selection bias by excluding from these analyses patients with "bad" recurrent disease who were deemed inoperable. The experienced RPS surgeon is likely to be very selective in choosing patients with recurrent RPS for attempted resection. Patient, treatment, and tumor factors (eg, obesity, debility, difficulty of the first operation, multifocal tumor, bone or major vascular involvement) that may not be readily captured in a published multivariable analysis will nonetheless be considered by the expert surgeon. These different factors may at least partially explain the discrepancies in the literature

Table 1
Margin status in retroperitoneal sarcoma series[a]

Author, Year	Number Resected	Primary Present[n] (%)	R0 n (%)	R1 n (%)	R2 n (%)	R Status Unknown n (%)	N.B.
Bonvalot et al,[21] 2010	249	100	R0/1:232 (93)		17 (7)		
Strauss et al,[22] 2010	200	100	55 (28)	85 (42)	30 (15)	30 (15)	170 known to have total gross resection (R0/1)
Sampath et al,[19] 2010	261	100	109 (42)	R1/2: 30 (11)		122 (47)	
Lehnert et al,[23] 2009	99	63	38 (38)	36 (36)	25 (25)		11 explored or biopsied only
Bonvalot et al,[9] 2009	374	100	176 (47)	103 (28)	38 (10)	57 (15)	8 biopsied only
van Dalen et al,[12] 2007	115	100	R0/1:78 (68)		37 (32)		8 explored only
Ballo et al,[17] 2007	83	72	44 (53)	R1/uncertain: 39 (47)			
Chiappa et al,[24] 2006	47	49	28 (60)	3 (7)	16 (33)		
Pierie et al,[15] 2006	103	100	R0/1:62 (60)		41 (40)		
Alldinger et al,[18] 2006	117	100	20 (17)	54 (46)	41 (35)	2 (2)	47 resected at outside institution
Erzen et al,[25] 2005	100	55	55 (55)	42 (42)	3 (3)		2 biopsied only
Zlotecki et al,[26] 2005	39	88	25 (64)	9 (23)	5 (13)		1 died preoperatively
Hassan et al,[38] 2004	89	100	R0/1:76 (85)		13 (15)		8 biopsied only
Gronchi et al,[16] 2004	167	49	R0/1:147 (88)		20 (12)		
Gilbeau et al,[28] 2002	45	100	17 (38)	26 (58)	2 (4)		
Jones et al,[29] 2002	46	65	R0/1:46 (100)		0		9 progressed preoperatively
Stoeckle et al,[14] 2001	145 M0	100	R0/1:94 (65)		Not available	Not available	20 had M1
Gieschen et al,[30] 2001	33	78	R0/1:29 (88)		4 (12)		4 no attempt to resect
Alektiar et al,[31] 2000	32	38	R0/1:30 (94)		2 (6)		

a 2000–2010; N.B, Nota Bene; N≥30.

with respect to the prognosis of patients with recurrent disease, which is generally inferior to that of those with primary RPS.

Compared with a 69% 5-year disease-specific survival rate[22] and a 57% 5-year overall survival rate[9] for primary RPS resection, the reported 5-year overall survival after R0/1 resection for recurrent RPS is much lower, at approximately 30%.[20] In the authors' own prospective study of multimodality radiation and surgery, disease-free and overall survivals were also significantly lower in the recurrent versus primary RPS subgroups.[29] In 70 patients with RPS (6 primary, 64 recurrent), most of whom were given intraoperative radiation, Dziewirski and colleagues[32] found that the patients with recurrent RPS had a 60% 2 year local recurrence–free survival rate (2-year disease-free survival was 58% in the authors' series) and a 75% 2-year overall survival rate (the authors' was 74%). These results emphasize that, even with limited follow-up, patients with recurrent RPS are quickly failing and dying of disease. Echoing these data, Ballo and colleagues[17] showed that 5-year local control rate was only 27% for resected recurrent RPS (n = 23) versus 58% for primary tumors (n = 60).

In contrast, two different studies showed that, although recurrent status was an independent predictor of worse local control and disease-free survival, it did not impact overall survival.[7,33] A group from Heidelberg[23] analyzed the outcomes of curative intent resection in 110 patients with RPS (71 primary, 39 recurrent cases) with a long median follow-up (89 months). Resectability rates, morbidity, and operative mortality were not different between the groups. However, 5-year local control was only 9% in the recurrent group compared with 59% in the primary group. Disease-specific survival rates after complete resection were comparable between the groups: 51% versus 43%, respectively. This phenomenon of multiple resections in highly selected patients with recurrent RPS (who eventually succumb to progressive disease or fatal operative complications, but only many years after their initial local recurrence) highlights selection bias as an important confounder of reported recurrent RPS outcomes. In a tri-institutional German series, Alldinger and colleagues[18] refer to this as an explanation for their finding that patients who had a local recurrence at some point in their disease course often had a better survival than those who never had local recurrence.

IMPROVING RPS OUTCOMES
Surgical Resection

Unanimous agreement exists that an RPS resection that leaves behind gross residual tumor is associated with reduced survival. The ability to achieve an R0/R1 resection can be enhanced by better patient selection, critical analysis of preoperative imaging, potential tumor downsizing with neoadjuvant therapy, and an improved intraoperative approach to resection.

Patient selection should include a detailed assessment of technical resectability combined with an appraisal of both physical and psychological risk tolerance. Selection is also contingent on a detailed review of good quality imaging by the operating surgeon. Failure to appreciate the extent of tumor, particularly with a well-differentiated liposarcoma, can lead to an inadvertent R2 resection (**Fig. 1**). Although RPSs are known for "pushing" rather than "infiltrative" margins, attachment to adjacent structures can be firm and vascular. Dense adherence to the wall of the IVC or aorta may necessitate en bloc resection even in the absence of clear invasion on imaging. The surgeon should be prepared to resect and reconstruct any organs that compose the perimeter of the tumor, including viscera, musculoskeletal, and major neurovascular structures. This resection might require participation by surgeons

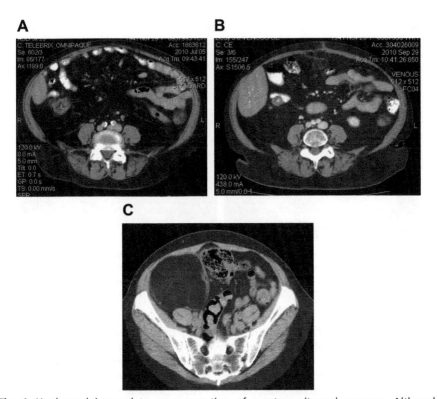

Fig. 1. Unplanned incomplete gross resection of a retroperitoneal sarcoma. Although preoperative imaging of this retroperitoneal liposarcoma was performed, the high-grade component adjacent to the descending colon (*A*) was not initially appreciated and was still present postoperatively (*B*). In another illustrative case, the postoperative image shown in (*C*) reveals a lack of appreciation for the low-grade component of this retroperitoneal liposarcoma; only the smaller high-grade component was resected by a general surgeon when consulted intraoperatively by a gynecologist.

from other subspecialties. Based on review of the imaging, the primary surgeon should plan for these possibilities, rather than compromising the resection because of a lack of available subspecialty expertise at the time of surgery. This approach to patient selection should yield a complete gross resection rate of close to 100%.[29]

Certain RPS subtypes may be responsive to neoadjuvant therapy, such as extraosseous Ewing's and primitive neuroectodermal tumor. In contrast, the predominant RPS histologies (liposarcoma and leiomyosarcoma) are not generally viewed as highly responsive to chemotherapy and/or RT. However, some authors have shown that a large RPS may decrease in size in response to neoadjuvant treatment.[34] In addition, there is anecdotal experience with significant downsizing of anatomically difficult, borderline resectable tumors, such as a large leiomyosarcoma of the IVC (**Fig. 2**). In these cases, neoadjuvant treatment could facilitate complete gross resection and, therefore, potentially improve local control. Although the data are limited, patients whose disease significantly progresses or whose performance status significantly declines on neoadjuvant therapy typically have a very poor prognosis.[29,35]

Although the value of complete gross resection is widely acknowledged, a lively debate exists among RPS specialists regarding two interrelated technical issues: the desirability/reality of R0 resection and an aggressive approach to surgical

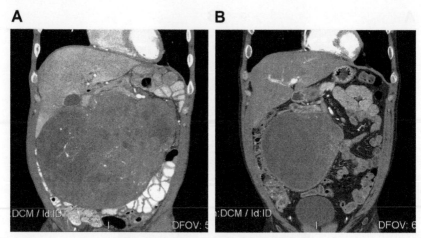

Fig. 2. Locally advanced leiomyosarcoma of the inferior vena cava. The tumor after three cycles of adriamycin/ifosfamide (*A*) and after subsequent completion of 25 fractions of radiation (*B*). The response to chemotherapy may not be immediately apparent on imaging, and chemotherapy/radiation may interact to effect preoperative downsizing.

resection. As noted in **Table 1**, the rate of R0 resection varies greatly in the literature. Anatomic constraints often preclude achieving 2-cm resection margins circumferentially around most RPS. However, en bloc resection of adherent organs seems advisable in light of evidence that most organs resected en bloc are microscopically infiltrated by tumor (Antonio Chiappa, MD, FACS, personal communication, 2011). Secondary questions then become "what is a reasonable quality of life 'price' for a patient to pay to achieve a microscopically negative margin?" and "is there value to achieving mostly negative margins circumferentially if one area will be microscopically positive?" Both questions are central to the arguments against the aggressive resection approach recently promulgated by several European centers.

The somewhat popular aggressive RPS resection movement has been led by both Gronchi and colleagues[7] in Milan and Bonvalot and colleagues[9] at the Institut Gustave-Roussy. In 2009, the *Journal of Clinical Oncology* published two large, retrospective series of RPS resections along with a cautionary editorial by Pisters.[36] The authors proposed a quasi-compartmental approach to RPS resection; for instance, advocating en bloc excision of the psoas muscle from its origins to insertion. The basis for the Italian argument was an improvement in local recurrence rates observed in a more recent cohort of patients undergoing the aggressive resection approach compared with historical controls. The shorter follow-up of the recent cohort was acknowledged. Bonvalot and colleagues[21] compared outcomes in contemporaneous cohorts of patients who underwent simple versus complete compartmental resection. On multivariate analysis, local control in the compartmental resection group was superior. However, the short-term morbidity in the French series was substantial, particularly an early reoperation rate of 8%. The morbidity associated with the compartmental approach in the Italian series was not addressed. Gronchi and colleagues[7] and Bonvalot and colleagues[9] subsequently combined their institutional experiences to focus on the safety of the aggressive approach, noting a major complication rate of 18%, an early reoperation rate of 12%, and a postoperative mortality of 3%. These rates are similar to reports by authors who use a more conventional, less aggressive resection strategy. Bonvalot and colleagues[9] and Gronchi and colleagues[7] also noted that morbidity increased with increasing numbers of organs resected en bloc with the tumor. Reassuringly, Tseng and colleagues[37] have shown that resection of contiguous organs is safe, at least in institutions participating in the American College of Surgeon National Surgical Quality Improvement Program. Issues of long-term morbidity related to unilateral nephrectomy and disorders of balance and movement related to neuro-muscular sacrifice have not been formally addressed.[38]

If one adopts a more pragmatic approach of preserving critical central retroperitoneal neurovascular and visceral structures to minimize morbidity (thereby compromising microscopic margin clearance), does that negate the value of resecting "disposable" organs/structures to obtain negative margins for most of the tumor's perimeter? Thomas and colleagues[22] at the Royal Marsden recently published their institutional experience with primary RPS resection. Essentially, surgery was performed by a limited number of highly experienced surgeons with the goal of complete gross tumor resection. Contiguous organs were resected if they appeared macroscopically involved, or to permit safe dissection, but adjacent organs that were clinically uninvolved were not resected. Although the median follow-up was relatively short at 29 months, the 5-year local recurrence–free and disease-specific survival rates were 55% and 75%, respectively, rivaling those published by Bonvalot and colleagues[9] and Gronchi and colleagues[7] for their aggressive surgical approach. Extrapolating from the literature on limb salvage extremity STS, one might also conclude that marginal excision along important neurovascular structures is appropriate. However, two important differences should be noted. First, death from extremity STS is overwhelmingly related to distant metastatic disease, whereas for RPS, it is most often from locoregional progression. Second, adjuvant RT has been shown to improve local control for extremity STS. The unclear role of RT for RPS is addressed in the next section.

Adjuvant RT

RT has a defined role in the treatment of STS, although most clinical trials have focused on extremity tumors. RT for RPS is less well established because of several factors. RPS is rare and the natural history can sometimes be indolent. Reports with less than 10 years of follow-up may provide an overly optimistic impression of the local control rates achieved with surgery alone. The sensitivity of critical abdominal viscera to radiation also places constraints on both the total dose and treatment volume that can be safely administered, particularly in the postoperative setting. This, in turn, limits the potential effectiveness of adjuvant RT to the point at which it has been offered to only select patients in many contemporary series.[12,16,18,19,21–23,27]

Most data regarding the efficacy of adjuvant RT for RPS come from population studies and secondary analyses of retrospective case series in which RT was used selectively.[6] Therefore, it is not surprising that the data are somewhat conflicting. Tseng and colleagues[6] noted no survival benefit to adjuvant RT in a SEER population-based registry of 1535 RPS cases. Only 373 patients (24%) received RT, with most (80%) in the postoperative setting. Sampath and colleagues[19] reported a significantly improved local failure-free survival for adjuvant RT in a cohort of 261 patients with primary RPS, although only 22% of patients actually received RT. Stoeckle and colleagues[14] also found significantly fewer local recurrences in the 61% of patients who received adjuvant RT in their cohort of 145 patients with primary RPS. Dziewirski and colleagues[31] found that significantly improved local control was associated with postoperative RT (external beam RT [EBRT] plus intraoperative RT [IORT]) in a cohort of 70 patients with RPS. However, median follow-up was only 20 months and 91% of patients had recurrent disease at presentation to their center.

Ballo and colleagues[17] and Gilbeau and colleagues[28] reported no advantage in local control associated with radiation dose-escalation with either EBRT or IORT. Gieschen and colleagues[30] noted a trend toward improved 5-year local control for 20 patients with RPS who received preoperative EBRT with IORT versus 9 patients treated with preoperative EBRT alone (68% vs 26%, $P = .068$). Most of the patients in the report (78%) were treated for a primary tumor presentation.

Complications from RT for RPS are not routinely reported in retrospective series. Zlotecki and colleagues[26] compared preoperative and postoperative RT in 40 patients with RPS and found that 80% of patients who received postoperative RT experienced acute enteritis versus only 36% who received preoperative RT ($P<.0098$). Ballo and colleagues[17] reported on late complications for 83 patients who underwent EBRT (preoperative in 50 patients, postoperative in 33 patients) with or without IORT. Clinically significant late radiation–related complications were identified in 5 patients (1 mild, 2 moderate, and 2 severe), all of whom received postoperative RT.

Gilbeau and colleagues[28] reported on 45 patients with RPS who received postoperative RT (28 patients had EBRT alone, 3 patients had IORT alone, 14 patients had IORT/EBRT). Moderate (grade 2) acute upper and lower gastrointestinal toxicity occurred in 45% and 30%, respectively. Severe and life-threatening (grade 3 and 4) acute gastrointestinal toxicity was seen in 2% and 5%, respectively. Fatal late gastrointestinal toxicity occurred in 2 patients. Peripheral sensory and motor neuropathy occurred in 8 patients (5 of whom received IORT). Gieschen and colleagues[30] reported on 37 patients treated with preoperative EBRT, with additional IORT administered to 20. All of the major late RT complications occurred in 4 of the 20 patients receiving IORT, including neuropathy, hydronephrosis, vaginal fistula, ureteroarterial fistula, and small bowel obstruction.

No randomized trials of adjuvant RT for RPS have been successfully completed, and only a limited number of prospective phase I/II trials have been performed. Pisters and colleagues[39] reported on a phase I trial to define the maximum tolerated dose of EBRT with concurrent doxorubicin for 35 patients with potentially resectable primary and recurrent high-grade RPS. This trial included neoadjuvant low-dose infusion doxorubicin chemotherapy with concurrent preoperative EBRT and an 18-Gy IORT boost. Preoperative RT was dose-escalated from 18 to 50.4 Gy in a stepwise fashion. Gross complete resection (R0 or R1) was performed in 26 of 29 patients. Grade 3 and 4 acute events were frequent (8 events in 11 patients) in the 50.4-Gy cohort. However, the multimodality regimen was believed to be feasible and safe at the 46.8- to 50.4-Gy level.

A prospective phase I/II trial by Jones and colleagues[29] examined EBRT plus postoperative brachytherapy in patients with primary or recurrent RPS. The planned total radiation dose was 70 Gy, with 45 to 50 Gy given as EBRT and 20 to 25 Gy as low-dose rate brachytherapy via catheters implanted at the time of surgery. The trial enrolled 55 patients, 9 of whom experienced progression or decline preoperatively and were not explored. R0/1 resection was achieved in 46 patients; EBRT was given preoperatively in 41 and postoperatively in 2. Brachytherapy was successfully administered in only 19 cases (upper abdominal application was abandoned later in the trial because of unacceptable toxicity). Four cases of grade 4 early postoperative toxicity and one grade 4 and two grade 5 late adverse events were associated with upper abdominal brachytherapy.

The 2-year disease-free and overall survival rates for resected patients were 80% and 88%, respectively. The authors concluded that the disease-free survival was promising and this approach warranted further investigation. However, brachytherapy to the upper abdomen was associated with significant morbidity and mortality, and subsequent tracking of late outcomes failed to reveal benefit.

Alektiar and colleagues[27] reported the results of a phase I/II trial of RPS surgical resection with 12- to 15-Gy high-dose rate intraoperative brachytherapy (IOBT) followed by postoperative EBRT in selected cases. Seventeen patients were excluded because of unresectability or technical problems with IOBT delivery. Postoperative EBRT was given to 78% (25/32) to a dose of 45 to 50.4 Gy. At a median follow-up of 33 months, the 5-year actuarial local control rate was 62%; 78% for primary presentation. Late complications were frequent and included gastrointestinal obstruction in 18%, fistula formation in 9%, peripheral neuropathy in 6%, hydronephrosis in 3%, and wound complications in 3%. As with the study by Jones and colleagues,[29] this trial showed the potential for high local control rates through combining surgery with RT, but with significant late toxicity from brachytherapy.

Newer high-precision EBRT techniques, such as image-guided intensity-modulated radiotherapy (IMRT), are particularly suited to treating retroperitoneal tumors when dose avoidance to normal viscera and radiation sensitive retroperitoneal structures is critical. Paumier and colleagues[40] performed a comparative RT planning study in which postoperative RT plans were generated and compared with IMRT and two different three-dimensional conformal treatment techniques. IMRT was believed to produce superior treatment plans with respect to overall radiation dose conformality, and also reduced volume of bowel that received 50 and 40 Gy, respectively. Bossi and colleagues[41] treated 18 patients with RPS with 50 Gy of preoperative IMRT, limiting the high-dose radiation treatment volume to the tumor–posterior abdominal wall interface (believed to be at the highest risk for local relapse). Treatment was well tolerated, with 3 patients developing grade 2 acute radiation-related gastrointestinal symptoms and only one experiencing grade 3 acute symptoms. Yoon and colleagues[42] reported on 28 patients who received highly conformed preoperative or postoperative EBRT using protons and/or IMRT. Preoperative treatment was used for 21 patients and IORT was given to 12 patients. Late RT complications occurred in 4 patients, including a ureteral stricture and an infected seroma in 2 patients who received IORT. Two patients who received IMRT required surgery; one for postoperative bleeding and another for a late enterocutaneous fistula. At a median follow-up of 33 months, local recurrence was seen in only 2 patients with a primary RPS (10%) versus 3 patients with a recurrent presentation (37.5%).

Systemic Chemotherapy

Given the challenges to and importance of obtaining local control in RPS, systemic chemotherapy has been considered as neoadjuvant cytoreductive therapy to improve R0 resectability for locally advanced disease, as a radiation sensitizer, or as definitive therapy for unresectable tumors. Sondak and colleagues[43] performed a prospective trial of the radiosensitizer idoxuridine with twice-daily preoperative RT for 57 patients with STS, including 20 with RPS. The planned RT dose for intraabdominal tumors was 62.5 Gy in 12.5-Gy fractions. Stomatitis was the dose-limiting toxicity for idoxuridine and 3 patients were taken off study. One patient with RPS had an objective response to treatment. At a median follow-up of 5.8 years, 5 local recurrences were seen in the 14 patients with RPS who ultimately underwent resection. Wendtner and colleagues[44] reported on a prospective series of 58 high-risk patients with locally advanced primary/recurrent RPS and visceral STS scheduled to receive four cycles of neoadjuvant etoposide, ifosfamide, and doxorubicin given with concomitant regional hyperthermia. Preoperative RT was also administered to previously unirradiated patients. Grade 4 nonhematologic toxicity occurred in 5 patients, and 2 patients died of sepsis during neoadjuvant therapy. Five partial and 8 minor treatment responses occurred. Thirty patients went on to surgical resection, which was R0 in 8 patients and R1 in

10. Local failure-free (59% vs 0%; *P*<.001) and overall survival rates (60% vs 10%; *P*<.001) significantly favored patients experiencing response to neoadjuvant radiation combined with a radiosensitizing agent. Any additional toxicity or benefit related to preoperative adriamycin could not be distinguished from that related to EBRT or IORT in the prospective dose-escalation trial reported by Pisters and colleagues.[39]

Centralized Multidisciplinary Care for RPS

Several authors have examined RPS treatment at high-volume centers with oncologic expertise versus lower-volume or community centers. van Dalen and colleagues[3] found a significantly lower rate of R2 resections at Memorial Sloan-Kettering Cancer Center (MSKCC) compared with a collection of multiple Dutch centers grouped together (18% vs 38%, respectively; *P* = .002). Survival was also better in patients managed at MSKCC, specifically for those with completely resected low-grade RPS with no distant metastases. Bonvalot and colleagues[9] found that the incidence of intraoperative tumor rupture inversely correlated with institutional volume. Not only the surgical approach varies among institutions; in an analysis of patients with RPS from the SEER database, Porter and colleagues[1] showed a significant regional variation in the use of RT. Pathologic analysis at centers of sarcoma expertise is also of critical importance.

There are data to support better RPS outcomes with management at a high-volume center. Analyzing 1722 patients with truncal sarcoma and RPS registered in the Florida Cancer Data System between 1981 and 2001, Gutierrez and colleagues[45] noted a significantly better overall survival for patients managed at a high-volume center. Over a 20-year period, Bonvalot and colleagues[9] found that institutional volume was a significant predictor of intraabdominal recurrence, with an adjusted hazard ratio of 1.61 if surgery occurred at a lower-volume center (defined as 10–30 RPS cases over 20 years). The correlation between volume and improved outcome may reflect a variety of processes of care, including a greater frequency of preoperative biopsy and multidisciplinary discussion.[9] Seinen and colleagues[2] found that the interval between initial referral and definitive management for patients with RPS treated in southern Sweden was longer at a specialized high-volume center. This interval reflected a longer investigational phase, which may be entirely appropriate given the broad differential diagnosis for a retroperitoneal mass and the importance of defining anatomic relationships in planning for complete gross tumor resection.

SUMMARY

Several factors have contributed to a lack of quality evidence regarding the optimal management of RPS, including its rarity, the tendency for patients to present with symptoms prompting urgent surgical intervention without substantive preoperative assessment, and the propensity for late recurrence necessitating very long-term follow-up to accurately assess disease control. The publication of large single- or multi-institutional retrospective series has provided a baseline against which to judge the results of future studies. Few prospective studies have been undertaken to date, and most have been small phase I/II trials. The authors applaud their European colleagues for initiating a European Organisation for Research and Treatment of Cancer (EORTC)–sponsored randomized trial of preoperative RT/resection versus resection alone for primary RPS. Pending the results of that trial, preoperative RT seems to have less toxicity than postoperative EBRT and may offer benefits in terms of both tumor targeting and normal tissue avoidance. Image-guided IMRT may provide further advantages for effective dose delivery, with lower toxicity to adjacent organs. The initial experience with this technique is encouraging. Ultimately, these important RT questions can only be definitively answered through appropriately designed, multicenter, prospective clinical trials. Many questions remain regarding the optimal management of recurrent RPS; treatment decisions should be made on a case-by-case basis. Finally, a starting point for documenting and improving RPS outcomes is consistent care by expert multidisciplinary teams working at high-volume centers.

REFERENCES

1. Porter G, Baxter N, Pisters P. Retroperitoneal sarcoma: a population-based analysis of epidemiology, surgery, and radiotherapy. Cancer 2006;106(7): 1610–6.
2. Seinen J, Almquist M, Styring E, et al. Delays in the management of retroperitoneal sarcomas. Sarcoma 2010;2010:702573.
3. van Dalen T, Hennipman A, Van Coevorden F, et al. Evaluation of a clinically applicable post-surgical classification system for primary retroperitoneal soft-tissue sarcoma. Ann Surg Oncol 2004;11:483–90.
4. Cheifetz R, Catton C, Kandel R, et al. Recent progress in the management of retroperitoneal sarcoma. Sarcoma 2001;5:17–26.
5. Lewis J, Leung D, Woodruff J, et al. Retroperitoneal soft-tissue sarcoma: an analysis of 500 patients treated and followed at a single institution. Ann Surg 1998; 228:355–65.
6. Tseng W, Martinez S, Do L, et al. Lack of survival benefit following adjuvant radiation in patients with retroperitoneal sarcoma: a SEER Analysis. J Surg Res 2011; 168(2):e173–8.
7. Gronchi A, Lo Vullo S, Fiore M, et al. Aggressive surgical policies in a retrospectively reviewed single-institution case series of retroperitoneal soft tissue sarcoma patients. J Clin Oncol 2009;27:24–30.
8. Catton C, O'Sullivan B, Kotwall C, et al. Outcome and prognosis in retroperitoneal soft tissue sarcoma. Int J Radiat Oncol Biol Phys 1994;29:1005–10.
9. Bonvalot S, Rivoire M, Castaing M, et al. Primary retroperitoneal sarcomas: a multivariate analysis of surgical factors associated with local control. J Clin Oncol 2009;27(1):31–7.
10. Singer S, Corson J, Demetri G, et al. Prognostic factors predictive of survival for truncal and retroperitoneal soft-tissue sarcoma. Ann Surg 1995;221: 185–95.
11. Alvarenga J, Ball AB, Fisher C, et al. Limitations of surgery in the treatment of retroperitoneal sarcoma. Br J Surg 1991;78:912–6.
12. van Dalen T, Plooij J, van Coevorden F, et al, Dutch Soft Tissue Sarcoma Group. Long-term prognosis of primary retroperitoneal soft tissue sarcoma. Eur J Surg Oncol 2007;33(2):234–8.
13. Nathan H, Raut C, Thornton K, et al. Predictors of survival after resection of retroperitoneal sarcoma: a population-based analysis and critical appraisal of the AJCC staging system. Ann Surg 2009;250:970–6.
14. Stoeckle E, Coindre JM, Bonvalot S, et al, French Federation of Cancer Centers Sarcoma Group. Prognostic factors in retroperitoneal sarcoma: a multivariate analysis of a series of 165 patients of the French Cancer Center Federation Sarcoma Group. Cancer 2001;92:359–68.
15. Pierie J, Betensky R, Choudry U, et al. Outcomes in a series of 103 retroperitoneal sarcomas. Eur J Surg Oncol 2006;32:1235–41.

16. Gronchi A, Casali P, Fiore M, et al. Retroperitoneal soft tissue sarcomas: patterns of recurrence in 167 patients treated at a single institution. Cancer 2004;100: 2448–55.
17. Ballo M, Zagars G, Pollock R, et al. Retroperitoneal soft tissue sarcoma: an analysis of radiation and surgical treatment. Int J Radiat Oncol Biol Phys 2007;67: 158–63.
18. Alldinger I, Yang Q, Pilarsky C, et al. Retroperitoneal soft tissue sarcomas: prognosis and treatment of primary and recurrent disease in 117 patients. Anticancer Res 2006;26(2B):1577–81.
19. Sampath S, Hitchcock Y, Shrieve D, et al. Radiotherapy and extent of surgical resection in retroperitoneal soft-tissue sarcoma: multi-institutional analysis of 261 patients. J Surg Oncol 2010;101(5):345–50.
20. Grobmyer S, Wilson J, Apel B, et al. Recurrent retroperitoneal sarcoma: impact of biology and therapy on outcomes. J Am Coll Surg 2010;210:602–10.
21. Bonvalot S, Miceli R, Berselli M, et al. Aggressive surgery in retroperitoneal soft tissue sarcoma carried out at high-volume centers is safe and is associated with improved local control. Ann Surg Oncol 2010;17(6):1507–14.
22. Strauss D, Hayes A, Thway K, et al. Surgical management of primary retroperitoneal sarcoma. Br J Surg 2010;97:698–706.
23. Lehnert T, Cardona S, Hinz U, et al. Primary and locally recurrent retroperitoneal soft-tissue sarcoma: local control and survival. Eur J Surg Oncol 2009;35(9): 986–93.
24. Chiappa A, Zbar A, Biffi R, et al. Effect of resection and outcome in patients with retroperitoneal sarcoma. ANZ J Surg 2006;76:462–6.
25. Erzen D, Sencar M, Novak J. Retroperitoneal sarcoma: 25 years of experience with aggressive surgical treatment at the Institute of Oncology, Ljubljana. J Surg Oncol 2005;91:1–9.
26. Zlotecki R, Katz T, Morris C, et al. Adjuvant radiation therapy for resectable retroperitoneal soft tissue sarcoma: the University of Florida experience. Am J Clin Oncol 2005;28(3):310–6.
27. Hassan I, Park SZ, Donohue JH, et al. Operative management of primary retroperitoneal sarcomas: a reappraisal of an institutional experience. Ann Surg 2004;239:244–50.
28. Gilbeau L, Kantor G, Stoeckle E, et al. Surgical resection and radiotherapy for primary retroperitoneal soft tissue sarcoma. Radiother Oncol 2002;65: 133–6.
29. Jones J, Catton C, O'Sullivan B, et al. Initial results of a trial of pre-operative external beam radiation therapy and post-operative brachytherapy for retroperitoneal sarcoma. Ann Surg Oncol 2002;9(4):346–54.
30. Gieschen H, Spiro I, Suit H, et al. Long-term results of intraoperative electron beam radiotherapy for primary and recurrent retroperitoneal soft tissue sarcoma. Int J Radiat Oncol Biol Phys 2001;50(1):127–31.
31. Alektiar K, Hu K, Anderson L, et al. High-dose-rate intraoperative radiation therapy (HDR-IORT) for retroperitoneal sarcomas. Int J Radiat Oncol Biol Phys 2000;47(1):157–63.
32. Dziewirski W, Rutkowski P, Nowecki Z, et al. Surgery combined with intraoperative brachytherapy in the treatment of retroperitoneal sarcomas. Ann Surg Oncol 2006;13(2):245–52.
33. Erzen D, Novak J, Spiler M, et al. Aggressive surgical treatment of retroperitoneal sarcoma: long-term experience of a single institution. Surg Technol Int 2007;16: 97–106.

34. Tzeng C, Fiveash J, Popple R, et al. Preoperative radiation therapy with selective dose escalation to the margin at risk for retroperitoneal sarcoma. Cancer 2006; 107:371–9.
35. Pawlik T, Pisters P, Mikula L, et al. Long-term results of two prospective trials of preoperative external beam radiotherapy for localized intermediate- or high-grade retroperitoneal soft tissue sarcoma. Ann Surg Oncol 2006;13:508–17.
36. Pisters P. Resection of some – but not all – clinically uninvolved adjacent viscera as part of surgery for retroperitoneal soft tissue sarcomas. J Clin Oncol 2009;27: 6–8.
37. Tseng W, Martinez S, Tamurian R, et al. Contiguous organ resection is safe in patients with retroperitoneal sarcoma: an ACS-NSQIP analysis. J Surg Oncol 2010;103(5):390–4.
38. Raut C, Swallow C. Are radical compartmental resections for retroperitoneal sarcomas justified? Ann Surg Oncol 2010;17:1481–4.
39. Pisters P, Ballo M, Fenstermacher M, et al. Phase I trial of preoperative concurrent doxorubicin and radiation therapy, surgical resection, and intraoperative electron-beam radiation therapy for patients with localized retroperitoneal sarcoma. J Clin Oncol 2003;21:3092–7.
40. Paumier A, Le Péchoux C, Beaudré A, et al. IMRT or conformal radiotherapy for adjuvant treatment of retroperitoneal sarcoma? Radiother Oncol 2011;99(1):73–8.
41. Bossi A, De Wever I, Van Limbergen E, et al. Intensity modulated radiation-therapy for preoperative posterior abdominal wall irradiation of retroperitoneal liposarcomas. Int J Radiat Oncol Biol Phys 2007;67(1):164–70.
42. Yoon S, Chen Y, Kirsch D, et al. Proton-beam, intensity-modulated, and/or intra-operative electron radiation therapy combined with aggressive anterior surgical resection for retroperitoneal sarcomas. Ann Surg Oncol 2010;17(6):1515–29.
43. Sondak V, Robertson J, Sussman J, et al. Preoperative idoxuridine and radiation for large soft tissue sarcomas: clinical results with five-year follow-up. Ann Surg Oncol 1998;5:106–12.
44. Wendtner C, Abdel-Rahman S, Krych M, et al. Response to neoadjuvant chemotherapy combined with regional hyperthermia predicts long-term survival for adult patients with retroperitoneal and visceral high-risk soft tissue sarcomas. J Clin Oncol 2002;20:3156–64.
45. Gutierrez J, Perez E, Moffat F, et al. Should soft tissue sarcomas be treated at high-volume centers? an analysis of 4205 patients. Ann Surg 2007;245:952–8.

Atypical Lipomatous Tumor/Well-Differentiated Liposarcoma: What Is It?

Melissa E. Hogg, MD[a], Jeffrey D. Wayne, MD[b],*

KEYWORDS

• Liposarcoma • Atypical lipomatous tumor • Sarcoma

According to the National Cancer Institute, soft tissue sarcomas (STSs) make up less than 1% of newly diagnosed cancers, with an incidence of 2.5 per million.[1] Liposarcoma (LPS) accounts for 24% of extremity and 45% of retroperitoneal STSs.[2] LPS often remains asymptomatic until quite large. When symptoms occur, they can be vague and frequently caused by mass effect.[1,3] LPSs can arise from any adipose tissue but are most commonly found in the thigh and retroperitoneum (**Fig. 1**). Like other STSs, prognosis varies depending on the site of origin, tumor size, depth, and grade. Recurrence rates range from 5% to 83%, with mortality rates from 1% to 90%.[4] First and foremost, the proper histologic classification is critical because this (along with tumor location) affects recurrence and survival. LPS has a diverse array of subclassifications; the biology is quite different and terminology can be controversial, confusing, and sometimes misleading.[5]

PATHOLOGIC CLASSIFICATION OF ADIPOCYTIC TUMORS

The pathologic classification of LPS in the overall spectrum of disease is represented by subtle nuances from low-grade to high-grade tumors, histologically classified based on their differentiation. Low-grade or well-differentiated LPS (WDLPS) consists of mature fat with the presence of lipoblasts, enlarged atypical nuclei, and clear multivacuolated cytoplasm and has been characterized by the amplification of

This work has no funding source.
The authors have nothing to disclose.
[a] Department of Surgical Oncology, University of Pittsburgh Medical Center, 5150 Centre Avenue, Suite 414, Pittsburgh, PA 15232, USA
[b] Melanoma and Soft Tissue Surgical Oncology, Division of Gastrointestinal and Oncologic Surgery, Department of Surgical Oncology, Northwestern University Feinberg School of Medicine, 676 North Saint Clair Street, Suite 650, Chicago, IL 60611, USA
* Corresponding author.
E-mail address: JWayne@nmff.org

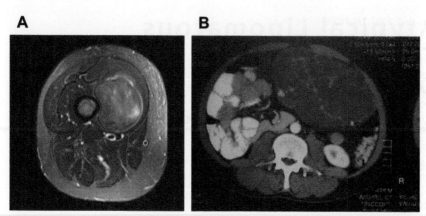

Fig. 1. Imaging modalities for LPS. (*A*) Magnetic resonance image of an extremity LPS. (*B*) Computed tomographic scan of a retroperitoneal LPS.

chromosome 12q 13–15.[2,5,6] Lipoblasts represent the hallmark of any malignant adipocytic tumor.[7]

Atypical lipomatous tumor (ALT) and WDLPS are sometimes synonymous terms used for a low-grade LPS and represent about 40% to 45% of all LPS.[8] Because WDLPS does not show metastatic potential unless associated with dedifferentiation and because wide excision is often curative, the term ALT was introduced. However, there is controversy regarding when this term is appropriate. Morphologically and genetically, ALT and WDLPS are identical.[9] Some investigators believe it is a pathologic diagnosis based on histology, others think it should be a combination of histology and anatomic location (eg, the extremity), and some suggest it should be reserved only for the appropriate histology and a clinically indolent course.[2,5,7,10]

On the other side of the biological spectrum, there are definitive criteria when an LPS should be classified as a dedifferentiated LPS (DDLPS): the presence of more than 5 mitotic figures per 10 high-power fields.[11] But tumor subclassification can be challenging because of the presence of fibrous tissue, myxoid tissue, varying degrees of cellularity, and lower numbers of mitotic figures. Problems with classification also arise when the tumor has more mitotic figures and cellularity than would be typical for a WDLPS diagnosis but less than for a DDLPS. Fibrous and/or myxoid zones can range from minimal to dominant. Some studies have expanded the subclassifications to form a spectrum between WDLPS and DDLPS such as a low-grade dedifferentiation category.[2,12,13] However, the true biological nature of this classification as being separate from WDLPS has yet to be proved.[6]

Evans[6] found that location and classification were the most important prognostic indicators for LPS; centrally based (deep) LPS and DDLPS had a worse prognosis than peripheral (superficial) LPS and WDLPS. These distinctions become important when counseling a patient on treatment, recurrence, metastatic risk, and survival. Low-grade variants have a 5-year survival of 90% versus survival rates for high-grade variants as low as 30% to 75%.[4] These tumors frequently recur, and a WDLPS can undergo dedifferentiation to become a DDLPS on recurrence.[6,12] The risk of dedifferentiation is time dependent and occurs approximately 20% of the time for retroperitoneal tumors and 5% for extremity tumors.[9] These rates increase with additional recurrences.[2]

CLINICAL EVALUATION OF WDLPS

Because LPS is rare, patients should be considered for referral to a multidisciplinary team with specific STS expertise.[14] All patients need to undergo imaging to determine tumor size, exact location, as well as contiguity or proximity to nearby critical structures. This is best accomplished by computed tomographic (CT) scan or magnetic resonance imaging (MRI). Both modalities have been shown to accurately predict tumor size and location relative to bone, joints, and neurovascular structures.[15] MRI can more accurately delineate anatomic compartments and muscle involvement. Therefore, it is thought to be better for extremity tumors. CT is preferentially used for central tumors (of the abdomen or retroperitoneum). It also provides very accurate information more rapidly and with less cost than MRI.[15,16]

Imaging characteristics have been described to differentiate WDLPS from DDLPS. Fat signal intensity is dominant in WDLPS. Conversely, imaging often reveals a heterogeneous nonlipogenic mass for DDLPS.[2] Imaging characteristics aside, a pathologic diagnosis is still necessary before planning treatment. Core needle biopsy is preferred, but, if unavailable or nondiagnostic, then an incisional biopsy along the long axis of the extremity is appropriate. Because neoadjuvant radiation or chemotherapy has not been conclusively shown to improve outcome for retroperitoneal WDLPS, preoperative biopsy remains controversial and is not imperative unless complete resection is not considered feasible.[2] Because STS, in general, preferentially metastasizes to the lungs, baseline cross-sectional chest imaging should be obtained. No other routine or special laboratory testing is required. A positron emission tomographic scan can be useful in certain circumstances but should not be used routinely in lieu of CT or MRI.[17,18]

SURGICAL RESECTION

Complete (R0) surgical resection provides the best chance for long-term relapse-free and overall survival. Thus, referring a patient with complex STS to a multidisciplinary team at a high-volume center is warranted.[14,19] The index surgery offers the best chance for cure, and the feasibility of subsequent operations is often diminished by altered anatomy, scar tissue, or sarcomatosis.[19] For extremity tumors, limb salvage surgery should be the goal. Patients should be referred to STS specialty centers before considering amputation.[20] Amputation is indicated if limb-sparing resection leaves grossly positive margins or a nonfunctional limb.[21–23] For intra-abdominal or retroperitoneal tumors, complete resection is achieved in only 50% to 95% of patients because of the proximity of vital structures.[19,24–28] However, complete resection still remains the most important factor affecting survival.[29] Specialty centers typically advocate a liberal en bloc resection but only with the goal and ability to achieve negative margins.[19,30] The quality of the surgical resection has been shown to be an independent risk factor for survival. Because of the high rates of local recurrence, retroperitoneal LPS can become a difficult management problem. This topic is discussed at length in other articles in this issue.

By and large, the earlier-mentioned recommendations are for all STSs; they are not specific for WDLPS alone. As previously mentioned, even the diagnosis of LPS represents a heterogeneous population of tumors. Retrospective STS studies include a large percentage of LPS; however, very few patients were specifically subclassified as having WDLPS or DDLPS. Therefore, the varying rates of distant metastases and survival seen in historical LPS series may reflect a failure to place WDLPS and DDLPS into separate subgroups. Regardless, WDLPS typically carries a more favorable prognosis because these patients often only develop locoregional recurrence, not systemic disease.[30] Anaya and colleagues[31] concluded that LPS, particularly WDLPS, is the only histologic STS subtype for which debulking might improve survival and provide palliation because of the low likelihood of metastases.[1] One study specifically addressing this issue found that surgical debulking can be effective for palliating symptoms and may also prolong survival, especially if surgery is the primary resection.[3] This is an obvious contradiction to general STS treatment recommendations but may be appropriate for highly selected cases of WDLPS. Thus, it may be argued that surgery should be considered in almost all patients presenting with a WDLPS.

THE ROLE OF RADIATION THERAPY

Although surgery is the primary treatment of WDLPS, adjuvant radiation may be considered in certain circumstances. Specifically, in the setting of an R1 resection or recurrent disease, adjuvant radiation therapy can be of benefit.[2,32] Although discussed at length by Delaney in another article in this issue, basic guidelines are as follows. A neoadjuvant approach is theoretically believed to be advantageous because it can sterilize the operative field and reduce recurrence risk due to less cellular shedding during tumor resection. Furthermore, because it does not need to include the entire operative bed, treatment fields are typically smaller.[33,34] Neoadjuvant radiation doses are typically 50 Gy for extremity, retroperitoneal, and intra-abdominal tumors.[35] The dosing of adjuvant therapy varies depending on the delivery method, final resection margin status, and history of previous radiation. At certain centers, intraoperative radiation therapy can be administered to areas thought to be at risk while sparing adjacent uninvolved tissues.

No randomized trials of adjuvant radiation for retroperitoneal WDLPS exist. Even retrospective studies have shown no proven survival benefit and only limited data to support a reduced risk for local recurrence.[1,36,37] In the absence of level 1 data, the potential role of multimodality therapy is left to best clinical judgment. Neoadjuvant radiation has theoretical advantages in intra-abdominal and retroperitoneal tumors because it may render unresectable or borderline resectable tumors more amenable to resection. The primary tumor also often displaces critical intra-abdominal organs out of the radiation field. Adjuvant radiation could be considered for an R0 resection of a DDLPS, an R0 resection of a WDLPS in the event of a large tumor and close margins, and all cases of R1 resection. However, the large volume of tissue to be irradiated with associated radiation injury to adjacent vital intra-abdominal organs often prohibits radiation therapy for retroperitoneal tumors.

RECURRENCE

The rate of recurrence for a central WDLPS is higher than that for an extremity tumor. A study of 92 WDLPS cases found that 91% of retroperitoneal tumors recurred versus only 43% of extremity tumors. In addition, the extremity tumors did not have any disease-specific mortality.[5] These investigators also noted that in 11 patients dedifferentiation occurred on recurrence. Evans[6] found that LPS, especially the retroperitoneal location and DDLPS histology, recurred frequently and often multiple times (usually <5 but up to 12 recurrences). When LPS recurs, it does not always have the same histologic classification as the original tumor. Frequently, WDLPS can recur as a DDLPS and even vice versa. The same holds true for subsequent recurrences. An important prognostic factor for retroperitoneal WDLPS and DDLPS is whether or not the tumor transformed when it recurred. Patients whose tumor became or remained a DDLPS had a worse outcome. Evans[6] found that only DDLPS, but never

WDLPS, metastasized hematogenously (median time, 44 months). The most common site was the lungs, but other organs included the liver, heart, pancreas, and spleen. Most patients with WDLPS died of recurrent disease. In essence, the clinical behavior of WDLPS and outcome strongly correlate with location.[6,12] Given the aggressive nature of retroperitoneal lipomatous tumors, some advocate only using the terminology WDLPS but not referring to these tumors as ALT because this could be clinically misleading.[5]

Local recurrence is best treated with resection. However, especially with retroperitoneal tumors, this can be difficult because of the proximity to vital structures and the frequency of recurrences. Some investigators have advocated clinical observation of a complex WDLPS recurrence because of the slow rate of growth combined with the potential morbidity associated with reresection.[2] One study calculated the growth rate of locally recurrent retroperitoneal LPS and found that only patients with growth rates less than 0.9 cm per month had improved survival after aggressive resection of the local recurrence.

SUMMARY

LPS represents a heterogeneous group of tumors with a large variability in malignant potential.[38,39] Given the rarity of LPS in general and the specific subclassifications in particular, little evidence is available to help delineate the best treatment strategy for WDLPS. What is apparent is that an overall biologically favorable prognosis has been demonstrated for WDLPS.[6,38,40] WDLPS may recur locally but rarely metastasizes systemically as the first site of disease recurrence. In a series of 1041 patients with extremity STS, non-LPS histology was an independent adverse prognostic factor for recurrence. However, this study did not differentiate between WDLPS and DDLPS. In another series, Gerrand and colleagues[41] found that only in 1 of 24 patients with WDLPS did the condition recur and no tumor metastasized. All patients were alive and disease free at a mean follow-up of 5 years. Given these results, some investigators have postulated that it is appropriate to accept a positive margin resection for WDLPS given its unique biological behavior. However, this strategy is controversial and has not been validated in the context of a clinical trial.

In a publication from Memorial Sloan Kettering Cancer Center, an attempt was made to develop treatment guidelines specific for WDLPS.[2] After surgical resection of an extremity LPS, adjuvant radiation was recommended for a DDLPS larger than 5 cm with close R0 or R1 resection margins. Chemotherapy was reserved only for patients with unresectable systemic disease. In contrast, this treatment algorithm was not recommended for an extremity WDLPS. For retroperitoneal LPS, systemic therapy was considered if surgery left gross tumor or the tumor growth rate of a local recurrence was more than 1 cm per month.[2]

Although a general consensus exists for the management of all STSs, this is not the case for WDLPS in particular. The favorable tumor biology associated with this histologic subtype may allow for a less aggressive treatment strategy for the primary tumor, but a more aggressive approach may be indicated in more advanced cases. Given the rarity of these tumors, patients with both ALT and WDLPS are better served by referral to a specialty center where pathologists, surgeons, medical oncologists, and radiation oncologists with expertise on STS can devise a multidisciplinary treatment plan based on the available data and clinical experience, while also accounting for the individual tumor biology and location.

REFERENCES

1. Neuhaus SJ, Barry P, Clark MA, et al. Surgical management of primary and recurrent retroperitoneal liposarcoma. Br J Surg 2005;92(2):246–52.
2. Crago AM, Singer S. Clinical and molecular approaches to well differentiated and dedifferentiated liposarcoma. Curr Opin Oncol 2011;23(4):373–8.
3. Shibata D, Lewis JJ, Leung DH, et al. Is there a role for incomplete resection in the management of retroperitoneal liposarcomas? J Am Coll Surg 2001;193(4): 373–9.
4. Dalal KM, Kattan MW, Antonescu CR, et al. Subtype specific prognostic nomogram for patients with primary liposarcoma of the retroperitoneum, extremity, or trunk. Ann Surg 2006;244(3):381–91.
5. Weiss SW, Rao VK. Well-differentiated liposarcoma (atypical lipoma) of deep soft tissue of the extremities, retroperitoneum, and miscellaneous sites. A follow-up study of 92 cases with analysis of the incidence of "dedifferentiation". Am J Surg Pathol 1992;16(11):1051–8.
6. Evans HL. Atypical lipomatous tumor, its variants, and its combined forms: a study of 61 cases, with a minimum follow-up of 10 years. Am J Surg Pathol 2007;31(1): 1–14.
7. Dei Tos AP. Liposarcoma: new entities and evolving concepts. Ann Diagn Pathol 2000;4(4):252–66.
8. Conyers R, Young S, Thomas DM. Liposarcoma: molecular genetics and therapeutics. Sarcoma 2011;2011:483154.
9. Coindre JM, Pedeutour F, Aurias A. Well-differentiated and dedifferentiated liposarcomas. Virchows Arch 2010;456(2):167–79.
10. Evans HL, Soule EH, Winkelmann RK. Atypical lipoma, atypical intramuscular lipoma, and well differentiated retroperitoneal liposarcoma: a reappraisal of 30 cases formerly classified as well differentiated liposarcoma. Cancer 1979;43(2):574–84.
11. Evans HL. Liposarcoma: a study of 55 cases with a reassessment of its classification. Am J Surg Pathol 1979;3(6):507–23.
12. Henricks WH, Chu YC, Goldblum JR, et al. Dedifferentiated liposarcoma: a clinicopathological analysis of 155 cases with a proposal for an expanded definition of dedifferentiation. Am J Surg Pathol 1997;21(3):271–81.
13. Elgar F, Goldblum JR. Well-differentiated liposarcoma of the retroperitoneum: a clinicopathologic analysis of 20 cases, with particular attention to the extent of low-grade dedifferentiation. Mod Pathol 1997;10(2):113–20.
14. Engstrom K, Bergh P, Gustafson P, et al. Liposarcoma: outcome based on the Scandinavian Sarcoma Group register. Cancer 2008;113(7):1649–56.
15. Demas BE, Heelan RT, Lane J, et al. Soft-tissue sarcomas of the extremities: comparison of MR and CT in determining the extent of disease. AJR Am J Roentgenol 1988;150(3):615–20.
16. Heslin MJ, Smith JK. Imaging of soft tissue sarcomas. Surg Oncol Clin N Am 1999;8(1):91–107.
17. Schuetze SM. Utility of positron emission tomography in sarcomas. Curr Opin Oncol 2006;18(4):369–73.
18. Schuetze SM, Rubin BP, Vernon C, et al. Use of positron emission tomography in localized extremity soft tissue sarcoma treated with neoadjuvant chemotherapy. Cancer 2005;103(2):339–48.
19. Lewis JJ, Leung D, Woodruff JM, et al. Retroperitoneal soft-tissue sarcoma: analysis of 500 patients treated and followed at a single institution. Ann Surg 1998; 228(3):355–65.

20. Rosenberg SA, Tepper J, Glatstein E, et al. The treatment of soft-tissue sarcomas of the extremities: prospective randomized evaluations of (1) limb-sparing surgery plus radiation therapy compared with amputation and (2) the role of adjuvant chemotherapy. Ann Surg 1982;196(3):305–15.

21. Williard WC, Collin C, Casper ES, et al. The changing role of amputation for soft tissue sarcoma of the extremity in adults. Surg Gynecol Obstet 1992;175(5): 389–96.

22. Ghert MA, Abudu A, Driver N, et al. The indications for and the prognostic significance of amputation as the primary surgical procedure for localized soft tissue sarcoma of the extremity. Ann Surg Oncol 2005;12(1):10–7.

23. Lin PP, Guzel VB, Pisters PW, et al. Surgical management of soft tissue sarcomas of the hand and foot. Cancer 2002;95(4):852–61.

24. Cody HS 3rd, Turnbull AD, Fortner JG, et al. The continuing challenge of retroperitoneal sarcomas. Cancer 1981;47(9):2147–52.

25. Kinsella TJ, Sindelar WF, Lack E, et al. Preliminary results of a randomized study of adjuvant radiation therapy in resectable adult retroperitoneal soft tissue sarcomas. J Clin Oncol 1988;6(1):18–25.

26. Jaques DP, Coit DG, Hajdu SI, et al. Management of primary and recurrent soft-tissue sarcoma of the retroperitoneum. Ann Surg 1990;212(1):51–9.

27. Karakousis CP, Velez AF, Gerstenbluth R, et al. Resectability and survival in retroperitoneal sarcomas. Ann Surg Oncol 1996;3(2):150–8.

28. Kilkenny JW 3rd, Bland KI, Copeland EM 3rd. Retroperitoneal sarcoma: the University of Florida experience. J Am Coll Surg 1996;182(4):329–39.

29. Heslin MJ, Lewis JJ, Nadler E, et al. Prognostic factors associated with long-term survival for retroperitoneal sarcoma: implications for management. J Clin Oncol 1997;15(8):2832–9.

30. Gronchi A, Lo Vullo S, Fiore M, et al. Aggressive surgical policies in a retrospectively reviewed single-institution case series of retroperitoneal soft tissue sarcoma patients. J Clin Oncol 2009;27(1):24–30.

31. Anaya DA, Lahat G, Wang X, et al. Postoperative nomogram for survival of patients with retroperitoneal sarcoma treated with curative intent. Ann Oncol 2010;21(2):397–402.

32. Eilber FC, Eilber FR, Eckardt J, et al. The impact of chemotherapy on the survival of patients with high-grade primary extremity liposarcoma. Ann Surg 2004; 240(4):686–95 [discussion: 95–7].

33. Yang JC, Chang AE, Baker AR, et al. Randomized prospective study of the benefit of adjuvant radiation therapy in the treatment of soft tissue sarcomas of the extremity. J Clin Oncol 1998;16(1):197–203.

34. Davis AM, O'Sullivan B, Bell RS, et al. Function and health status outcomes in a randomized trial comparing preoperative and postoperative radiotherapy in extremity soft tissue sarcoma. J Clin Oncol 2002;20(22):4472–7.

35. NCCN Soft Tissue Sarcoma Guidelines, v2.2011, Guidelines for Radiation Therapy. Available at: www.nccn.org. Accessed November 29, 2011.

36. Mendenhall WM, Zlotecki RA, Hochwald SN, et al. Retroperitoneal soft tissue sarcoma. Cancer 2005;104(4):669–75.

37. Pawlik TM, Pisters PW, Mikula L, et al. Long-term results of two prospective trials of preoperative external beam radiotherapy for localized intermediate- or high-grade retroperitoneal soft tissue sarcoma. Ann Surg Oncol 2006;13(4):508–17.

38. Zagars GK, Goswitz MS, Pollack A. Liposarcoma: outcome and prognostic factors following conservation surgery and radiation therapy. Int J Radiat Oncol Biol Phys 1996;36(2):311–9.

39. Ng YC, Tan MH. Liposarcoma of the extremities: a review of the cases seen and managed in a major tertiary hospital in Singapore. Singapore Med J 2009;50(9): 857–61.
40. Chang HR, Gaynor J, Tan C, et al. Multifactorial analysis of survival in primary extremity liposarcoma. World J Surg 1990;14(5):610–8.
41. Gerrand CH, Wunder JS, Kandel RA, et al. Classification of positive margins after resection of soft-tissue sarcoma of the limb predicts the risk of local recurrence. J Bone Joint Surg Br 2001;83(8):1149–55.

Sarcomas and the Immune System: Implications for Therapeutic Strategies

Valerie Francescutti, MD[a], Joseph J. Skitzki, MD[a,b],*

KEYWORDS

• Sarcoma • Immunotherapy • Antigen • Vaccine
• Immunoediting

Sarcomas are rare tumors that account for less than 1% of all adult cancers.[1] The role of the immune system in cancer was first studied in sarcomas as immune responses to a bacterial toxin challenge were observed in metastatic bone sarcoma patients. Instances of spontaneous sarcoma regression and the observation of immune responses in human immunodeficiency virus (HIV) patients with Kaposi sarcoma undergoing antiretroviral therapy further suggest an immune-mediated antisarcoma mechanism. The development of sarcoma cell lines in preclinical animal models has allowed for further investigation of immune-related therapies, leading to clinical trials in sarcoma vaccines and cellular adoptive immunotherapy. Important to this burgeoning field, the discovery of tumor-associated antigens (TAAs) specific to sarcoma has been critical for the continued development of targeted therapies.

This review highlights the early studies of the immune system and its relationship to sarcomas, preclinical models designed to study the immunology of sarcomas, and the most current immunotherapy trials in the field. As a group, these tumors are generally thought of as aggressive, with high rates of mortality secondary to metastatic disease.[2] As the prognosis for metastatic sarcoma is generally poor, an improved understanding of and the ability to manipulate the immune system is emerging as a viable treatment modality.[3]

The authors have nothing to disclose.
[a] Department of Surgical Oncology, Roswell Park Cancer Institute, Elm and Carlton Streets, Buffalo, NY 14263, USA
[b] Department of Immunology, Roswell Park Cancer Institute, Elm and Carlton Streets, Buffalo, NY 14263, USA
* Corresponding author. Department of Surgical Oncology, Roswell Park Cancer Institute, Buffalo, NY 14263.
E-mail address: joseph.skitzki@roswellpark.org

Surg Oncol Clin N Am 21 (2012) 341–355
doi:10.1016/j.soc.2011.11.002
1055-3207/12/$ – see front matter © 2012 Elsevier Inc. All rights reserved.

HISTORICAL PERSPECTIVE

In an indirect fashion, immune responses to cancer were first noted in sarcoma, dating back to 1891, by the bone sarcoma surgeon, William B. Coley.[4] Coley conducted a series of experiments based on his clinical experience of patients with metastatic sarcoma and reports of infections causing tumor regression. Searching for better treatment options, he became aware of a sarcoma patient who had previously failed multiple surgical resections and who then developed a high fever due to an erysipelas infection followed by an unexpected regression of his large tumor burden. Therefore, Coley proposed and performed the injection of live streptococcal organisms directly into the tumors of patients with bone sarcoma in the hope of recapitulating the previously observed findings.[5] These initial treatments proved to be fatal in two patients, though some decrease in primary tumor size was noted.[6] Further experiments were completed using heat-inactivated streptococcal organisms, along with *Serratia marcescens*; the combination was named Coley's Toxin or Erysipelas Toxin. Over the next 20 years, Coley's Toxin was used to treat patients who had mainly inoperable sarcomas of the bone or soft-tissue sarcomas (STS). Not only was shrinkage of the primary tumor observed, but metastatic lesions also were found to be similarly responsive. This finding led Coley to hypothesize that a systemic phenomenon was responsible. During this period, Coley's work was criticized by a skeptical medical community because of the inconsistencies related to patient follow-up, method of administration of the toxin, and different available preparations.[7] Coley's daughter, however, continued this line of investigation and analyzed more than 1000 cases treated by Coley's Toxin, with approximately 500 partial to complete responses.[8] Subsequently a controlled study was undertaken in 1962, showing a response in 20 of 93 (21.5%) patients.[9] By this time, the use of Coley's Toxin had fallen out of favor for the treatment of sarcomas, due to the emergence of radiation as a standard therapy with more predictable toxicities.

Coley's contributions to cancer immunotherapy were profound, albeit indirect, and laid the groundwork for ongoing immunologic approaches. For example, the underlying mechanism of Coley's Toxin was found to be primarily related to bacterial endotoxin effects on the tumor-bearing host.[9] Discovered in the 1970s, it was thought that tumor necrosis factor α (TNF-α) may have been the major host mediator of Coley's Toxin.[10] While TNF-α demonstrated overlapping toxicities to Coley's Toxin, it did not produce the same degree of antitumor activity. Furthermore, the use of TNF-α to generate antitumor responses required the presence of tumor-sensitized immune cells. Similarly, Coley's Toxin appeared to work best in patients with immunogenic tumors and in patients with preexisting immunity. As a multitude of cytokines have been discovered since that time, there are data to support interleukin-12 (IL-12) as a likely mediator of Coley's Toxin.[11] Unfortunately, systemic use of IL-12 is associated with prohibitive toxicities, so efforts to localize delivery of IL-12 to tumors are currently being explored.

Evidence for Immunoediting and an Immune Response in Sarcomas

Theories of the host immune system being capable of shaping the development, outgrowth, and potential responses to growing tumors has been increasingly accepted, and are applicable to sarcomas (**Table 1**). The initial theory of immunosurveillance was formally introduced by Burnet and Thomas in 1957, stating that one of the main functions of cellular immunity was to protect from neoplastic change.[12] In recent years, Schreiber has further championed and expanded this theory of "immunoediting" and is supported by a growing body of experimental results.[13] As an

Table 1
Evidence for immune response in sarcoma

	Immune Response	Comment
Host response	Lymphocytic infiltration of tumor	Infiltration of primary tumor with lymphocytes associated with improved survival[17–19]
	Spontaneous regression	Seen in desmoids tumors most frequently, especially in the postpartum period[20,21] Case reports of spontaneous regression in other sarcoma types including osteosarcoma[22]
	Unplanned resections	Incomplete resection occurs at first surgery with repeat excision for positive margins yielding no further tumor[23] and improved outcomes[24]
Sarcoma-specific antigenicity	Antibody cross-reactivity in sarcoma patients	Antibodies from one sarcoma patient cross-reacts to sarcomas from different patients, with similar and dissimilar histologies[28,29]
	Immunization with irradiated sarcoma cells	Injection of patients with their own irradiated sarcoma cells results in rising cytotoxic antibody titers[30]
Viral	Kaposi sarcoma	In human immunodeficiency virus patients with Kaposi sarcoma (KS), caused by human herpesvirus 8 (HHV8), initiation of highly active antiretroviral therapy is associated with an increase in CD4$^+$ counts, and partial or complete regression of KS lesions, with a decrease in HHV8 viral load[33–35]

encompassing term, immunoediting is responsible for eliminating neoplastic cells and determining the immunologic phenotypes of tumors that form.[11–14] There are 3 accepted phases of immunoediting that occur as a spontaneous cancer cell arises; elimination, equilibrium, and escape.[15] The elimination phase depicts an immune system capable of recognizing and destroying aberrant cancer cells, which is likely a frequent event. In the less common equilibrium phase, cancer cells are able to evade initial destruction and maintain a balance with the immune system under selection pressures to avoid elimination. In the escape phase, tumor growth and metastases are no longer controlled by the immune system. This final phase represents growth of cancer cells that have acquired the ability to avoid immune-system detection by a variety of means that are a compilation of adaptive changes. While it would be intuitive to assume that the process of immunoediting is governed by the adaptive arm of the immune system, there is evidence of innate immunity being capable of sculpting tumor evolution as well.[16] Germane to this discussion, Schreiber had initially demonstrated many of the principles of immunoediting in murine models of sarcoma.[17] Similar to these murine models, there are several lines of clinical evidence showing endogenous host immune responses to have a role in the immunoediting of sarcoma.[13]

Lymphocytic infiltration of tumors, indicating an immune response, has been associated with improved patient survival.[18] This observation has been recently reported in patients with Ewing sarcoma, as the number of tumor-infiltrating CD8[+] T lymphocytes was directly correlated with improved survival as opposed to CD8[+] T lymphocytes found in the surrounding stroma.[19] Furthermore, infiltrating cytotoxic CD8[+] T lymphocytes were linked with the detection of proinflammatory cytokine attractants or chemokines expressed by the tumors, suggesting a causal mechanism. Conversely, if high concentrations of T-regulatory cells are found in the bone marrow of Ewing sarcoma patients, this has been associated with metastatic disease.[20] These T-regulatory cells, defined by the phenotype of $CD4^+CD25^{hi}FoxP3^+$, are known inhibitors of cytotoxic CD8[+] T lymphocytes and likely promote tumor escape with subsequent metastases.

Additional evidence for a host antitumor immune response includes spontaneous tumor regression. Spontaneous regression has been typically reported in tumors such as cutaneous melanoma and renal cell carcinoma. Although spontaneous regression in sarcoma is rare, it is occasionally seen in desmoid tumors or fibromatosis following hormonal changes associated with the postpartum state.[21,22] There are also reports of partial spontaneous regression with lymphocyte infiltration of extraskeletal osteosarcoma, supporting a role for the immune system in this process.[23] Of interest is that following unplanned resections of extremity soft-tissue tumors that are found to be a positive-margin STS on final pathology, re-resection yields residual disease in only 35% of patients. These findings further support the possibility of a host immune response to sarcoma.[24] A large analysis of extremity STS patients at Memorial Sloan-Kettering Cancer Center reported by Lewis and colleagues[25] also demonstrates a potential immune-mediated component to sarcoma outcome. A total of 685 primary extremity STS patients who underwent initial definitive resection were compared with 407 similar patients treated with a definitive reexcision following a previous nontherapeutic excision at an outside institution. Unexpectedly, the 5-year disease-free survival for the definitive versus re-resected patients was significantly different, at 70% versus 88%, respectively ($P = .0001$). These survival differences could not be explained by a referral bias, which would presume that more advanced or complicated patients would be seen at a tertiary center that could provide a single definitive surgery. In fact, when analyzed according to stage, all re-resected patients trended toward an improved outcome in comparison with the definitively treated group, which was statistically significant ($P = .005$) for the stage III group (>5 cm, deep, high grade) These observations extended beyond the local recurrence-free survival, as there was also an improvement in metastasis-free survival for the re-resected group, suggesting a possible systemic effect. Given these observations in extraskeletal osteosarcomas and primary extremity STS, it can be postulated that an incomplete initial excision may prime an immune response against remaining tumor cells, leading to improved residual tumor-cell elimination or equilibrium.

The loss of major histocompatibility complex I (MHC I) on sarcoma cells is seen as a means of escaping immune-system elimination. All nucleated cells express MHC I on their cell surface, which acts as a marker for recognition by the cellular arm of the immune system. Foreign antigens, such as viral proteins, can be presented on MHC I molecules and recognized by CD8[+] T cells, leading to efficient killing of the infected cell. In a parallel fashion, unique tumor antigens may be expressed on

MHC I molecules found on the tumor cell surface, which can lead to elimination of the tumor cell by CD8$^+$ T cells. There is a substantial body of literature addressing tumor loss of MHC I molecule expression as a means of escaping recognition by the immune system.[26] In a study concerning sarcomas specifically, MHC I was lost or downregulated in 46 of 74 (62%) various histologic types.[26] Patients with osteosarcoma that expressed MHC I had a significantly better overall and event-free survival than those with MHC I–negative osteosarcoma, suggesting the importance of cellular immunologic responses to sarcoma.

Humoral or antibody immune responses to sarcomas were shown by Mitchell[27] and Morton[28] in a series of patients with a variety of soft-tissue and bone sarcomas. Antigenicity appeared to be common and nonspecific among all the sarcomas studied, as fluorescein-conjugated antibodies from patients with one type of sarcoma were found to cross-react in vitro against tumors with both similar and dissimilar histologies.[29,30] However, an immune response specific to a particular tumor was shown to be generated in the sarcoma-bearing host, as antibodies found in the serum could be used to identify circulating or excreted sarcoma antigens in the same patient's urine.[31] These observations indicate that a common antigenicity may exist between sarcomas, regardless of histology, and that an immune response specific to a particular sarcoma is identifiable in individual patients.

To test this immune-response concept, Gupta and Morton[31] collected 24-hour urine samples from sarcoma patients, both before and after surgical resection. Serum was also collected 2 weeks after resection when sarcoma antibody titers were found to be highest. The antigenic activity of urine and serum was tested using the ultra-microcomplement fixation test. Urine and serum samples from healthy volunteers did not show any reactivity against tumor cells, whereas urine and serum samples from 12 of 13 sarcoma patients reacted positively against autologous and allogeneic sarcoma serum. Reactivity of the urine to sarcoma sera disappeared after surgical ablation of the tumor mass and reappeared following clinical recurrence of the tumor in 2 patients. This study demonstrated that sarcoma-specific antigens were present in both the serum and urine of sarcoma patients, and that specific antibody titers varied with tumor volume.

Further insight into the immune response to sarcoma can be found in immunosuppressed patients with Kaposi sarcoma (KS). Human herpesvirus 8 (HHV8) or KS-associated herpesvirus (KSHV) is the known causative oncogenic virus for KS, which in general portends a poor prognosis.[32] Clinical KS can be grouped into 4 epidemiologic forms: classic KS affecting men of eastern European Jewish background, endemic KS occurring in Central and East Africa, iatrogenic KS developing in immunosuppressed patients after organ transplant, and epidemic or AIDS-KS, a major AIDS-defining malignancy in the Western world.

In the HIV-infected population, KS is the most common neoplasm of untreated individuals.[32] Once highly active antiretroviral therapy (HAART) was introduced, a decline in the incidence of KS was observed in the HIV-positive population.[33] The reason for this unexplained decrease in KS incidence was hypothesized to be related to improvement in the host's immune system, thereby allowing for an immune response against the virally induced sarcoma. To further elucidate the reason for this unexplained decrease in incidence, a prospective study was undertaken to monitor immune responses of HIV-positive patients with identified KSHV infection while receiving HAART. Following 52 weeks of HAART treatment, decreases in both HIV-1 and KSHV titers were noted, which were associated with significant increases in CD4$^+$ T-lymphocyte counts.[34] In a further study, 29 patients with HIV infection, 21 with KS and 8 without KS, were evaluated prospectively during HAART. Nearly half of the patients with KS had a favorable response to HAART, with a complete clinical response/remission in 6 patients and a partial response (defined as shrinkage of the primary KS) in 4 patients. Of the 20 patients with detectable KSHV viral load before the initiation of HAART, 60% had undetectable viral loads with therapy.[35] These studies confirm that sarcoma responses can be directly related to the status of the host's immune system.

Preclinical Data for Sarcoma Immunotherapy

A series of preclinical studies completed in the 1980s were some of the first to lay the groundwork for immunotherapy for sarcoma in humans. By this time, methylcholanthrene-induced fibrosarcoma (meth A) cell lines had been well established as a model of syngeneic transplantable sarcomas in mice.[36] Meth A–implanted tumors grew progressively and were lethal to the host. However, when meth A tumor cells were injected jointly with a mixture of formalin-killed *Propionibacterium acnes* bacteria, tumors grew for 9 days and would then spontaneously reject. The tumor rejection was found to be a T-cell–mediated phenomenon, and the antitumor immunity of these cured mice could be transferred into other meth A tumor-bearing mice. To transfer this immunity, the tumor-bearing hosts had to either be lethally irradiated/restored with bone marrow or undergo immunosuppression with cyclophosphamide before receiving donor T cells from the cured mice. The transferable immunity was limited in that it was incapable of treating tumors that were established for more than 9 days.[37] This ability to generate and transfer antitumor immunity in preclinical models is a cornerstone of current adoptive immunotherapy protocols.

In similar animal models developed at the National Cancer Institute, mouse fibrosarcomas were generated by injecting methylcholanthrene (MCA) intramuscularly, and malignant cells harvested for tissue culture. The 2 main tumor types, MCA 105 and MCA 106, were used to dissect issues of adoptive immunotherapy. Similar to the meth A sarcoma studies, adoptive transfer of spleen cells from mice immunized with MCA 105 or MCA 106 tumor cells induced complete regression of existing MCA 105 and MCA 106 fibrosarcomas in host mice, respectively.[38] As a more stringent model, the MCA series of sarcoma tumors were used within the first 5 transplantation passages so that the tumor-associated transplantation antigens were more representative of the initial tumor, without genetic alteration. Further characterization of the effector cells generated after stimulation with MCA 105 cells showed that regression of the preestablished MCA 105 sarcoma was done in an antigen-specific fashion.[39] These studies served as the basis for the process by which lymphocytes from sarcoma-bearing mice could be expanded and sensitized, using an in vitro sensitization procedure and expansion with interleukin-2 (IL-2).[40] The ability to eradicate established MCA sarcoma pulmonary metastases by adoptive transfer of activated and expanded lymphocytes has been well reported.[41–43]

More recent preclinical studies have used cytokines historically associated with sarcoma regression to target the tumor microenvironment and enhance endogenous immune responses. Using the MCA 205 sarcoma line, TNF-α and IL-12 delivery by a slow-release mechanism has demonstrated significant antitumor effects.[44] The mechanism of action seems to be dependent on cytotoxic T cells and natural killer (NK) cells. Intratumoral treatment of a primary MCA 205 tumor with TNF-α and IL-12 led to growth inhibition of synchronous subcutaneous tumors or pulmonary metastases, which was abrogated by the depletion of endogenous T cells or NK cells. Furthermore, the antitumor lymphocytes generated from this approach were able to be transferred into mice bearing similar MCA 205 tumors and to mediate significant tumor regression of established pulmonary metastases. The ability of IL-12 to enhance immune responses has also been demonstrated in murine models of sarcoma vaccines.[45] In addition, gene-transfer protocols for the delivery of IL-12 have been developed in murine sarcoma models, and show antitumor synergy with radiation.[46] These preclinical studies demonstrate the ability to localize cytokines or deliver synergistic doses, which are normally toxic when given systemically, to create antisarcoma immune responses. Collectively these studies strongly support the clinical application of cellular immunotherapy for sarcoma, and are a basis for clinical trials.

In terms of a humoral approach, the development of monoclonal antibodies (MoAb) led to the theory that immunotherapy by passive administration of antibodies to patients with sarcomas might be a simple and effective therapy. This concept was tested through a series of preclinical studies in a murine sarcoma model. MoAb directed against Moloney sarcoma cells (MSC) were produced by fusion of spleen cells to antibody-producing cells. BALB/c mice with existing sarcomas were given 3 schedules of antibody injection; MoAb injected prior to sarcoma tumor-cell inoculation, on the same day of inoculation, and 4 days after the establishment of sarcoma tumor. MoAb injection was found to significantly prolong the life span of all mice, regardless of the injection regimen. However, MoAb given to mice with very large tumors (>10 days after implantation) did not prolong survival significantly.[47] This model also was used to test factors affecting passive MoAb therapy. In evaluating the mechanism underlying the improved survival in MSC-bearing mice treated with MoAb, nu/nu mice, those depleted of complement, and mice that were irradiated before treatment all showed a response to MoAb treatment. This finding indicated that the MoAb therapy effect was independent of complement, B cells, or cytotoxic T-cell responses, and may indicate direct antibody-mediated cell lysis.[48]

CLINICAL DATA FOR SARCOMA IMMUNOTHERAPY
Vaccines

Vaccines directed against tumor-specific peptides, proteins, and DNA have shown varying degrees of success in the treatment of cancer.[49] Vaccine strategies for the treatment and prevention of sarcoma recurrence are intriguing as they represent a targeted, tumor-specific, nontoxic therapy. Sarcomas are ideal vaccine targets, as tumor tissue can often be obtained in abundance for the generation of a variety of vaccines. The potential for repeated and late sarcoma recurrence, particularly in the case of retroperitoneal liposarcomas, also makes a preventive-vaccine approach attractive.

In clinical terms, vaccine treatment for sarcoma dates back to the 1960s with a whole-cell and cell-lysate sarcoma vaccine for osteogenic sarcoma.[40] In postamputation patients, encouraging responses to cell-lysate vaccine therapy were noted, with the primary end point being a delay in the development of pulmonary metastases.[50,51] Although this early study was weakened by its reliance on historical controls for comparison, it highlighted a standardized method for vaccine generation and clinical delivery. A more recent study of a vaccine derived from an autologous tumor cell line demonstrated the feasibility of establishing a short-term culture of human sarcoma cells followed by irradiation and cryopreservation for use in a subcutaneous vaccination protocol.[52] Delayed-type hypersensitivity (DTH) reactions were monitored during the vaccination period, which consisted of weekly injections for 3 weeks followed by monthly injections for 5 months. In this trial vaccine was successfully generated from 56% of the patients, and DTH responses were noted in half of the vaccinated patients by week 3. Although no objective antitumor responses were observed, this study provided encouraging findings regarding vaccine generation, safety, and potential immune readouts in sarcoma patients.

Some novel vaccine approaches have already been investigated for tolerability and immune responses. For example, osteosarcoma overexpresses a glycoprotein designated CD55, which protects from immune complement attack.[53] This overexpression was exploited as a potential target for a clinical trial of immune therapy in patients with metastatic osteosarcoma or those having a high risk of recurrence. Following 1 to 6 months of myelosuppressive chemotherapy, patients were vaccinated with an anti-idiotypic antibody to mimic CD55 in an attempt to generate immunity against tumor-expressed CD55. The majority of patients in this trial showed measurable T-helper cell responses as evidenced by increased T-cell proliferation and interferon-γ secretion, while no significant toxicity was noted.[54]

Contemporary vaccine immunotherapies have used dendritic cells (DC), which act as antigen-presenting cells in vivo.[55] DCs can sensitize T cells to tumor-specific antigens and induce cytotoxic T lymphocytes.[56] This approach was applied in a study of pediatric patients with relapsed solid tumors, a large percentage of which were sarcomas. DCs were generated from peripheral blood samples from these patients and were pulsed with tumor-cell lysates ex vivo. Tumor-cell lysates are thought to prime DCs to present a variety of tumor-associated antigens. Intradermal injection of 1×10^6 or up to 1×10^7 tumor-lysate pulsed DCs was performed every 2 weeks for a total of 3 injections. Pediatric patients with Ewing sarcoma, osteosarcoma, and fibrosarcoma were treated, and significant tumor regression was noted in the metastatic fibrosarcoma patient.[57] The study demonstrated that a DC vaccine protocol could be completed safely and with minimal toxicity in an outpatient setting.

As an example of targeting a specific translocation mutation found in sarcoma, a DC vaccine protocol was used in an 11-year-old patient with relapsed synovial sarcoma. DCs were generated from peripheral blood and were pulsed with a peptide from the SYT-SSX fusion protein commonly found in synovial sarcoma cells. The vaccination with sensitized DCs was well tolerated and arrested the growth of lung metastases for 4 months.[58] In a pilot study of 52 pediatric patients with metastatic or recurrent Ewing sarcoma or alveolar rhabdomyosarcoma, patients underwent immune cell harvest, standard chemotherapy, and immune therapy involving autologous T cells and DCs pulsed with peptides derived from tumor-specific translocation break points. Toxicity was minimal and the 5-year overall survival rate was 43%, comparing favorably with results in the literature.[59]

Use of Adjuvants

The use of adjuvants, or agents designed to enhance the activity of vaccines without any antigenic effect itself, have also been investigated. Recent developments in this area include the concept of costimulation, whereby the immune response from a vaccine can be made more effective by providing stimulation of immune-specific T cells.[60] In vitro studies indicate that granulocyte macrophage-colony stimulating factor (GM-CSF) is a powerful immunostimulant, and that the host response to a tumor can be amplified by vaccination with tumor cells altered to express GM-CSF.[61] In a phase I study of GM-CSF gene-transfected autologous sarcoma cells, the technique was deemed safe and feasible in a vaccine protocol. Unfortunately only a small number of patients, 4 of 17 (23.5%), had a clinically elevated level of gene expression.[62] A comparative phase II trial of autologous tumor vaccine with either adjuvant interferon-γ or adjuvant GM-CSF for solid tumors included STS patients with advanced or metastatic disease. Both adjuvants were well tolerated. Five-year overall survival was 25%, with minimal differences between the two arms.[52] In another vaccine study of patients with recurrent Ewing sarcoma or alveolar rhabdomyosarcoma, immature dendritic cells were pulsed with peptides derived from break-point regions of tumor-specific fusion proteins. As an adjuvant, patients received a concurrent intravenous infusion of IL-2. Toxicity was mild and was mostly related to the known adverse effects of IL-2. The peptide vaccination and IL-2 combination in this study did not alter the clinical outcomes for these patients, as only one patient showed evidence of an immunologic response.[63]

The search for natural adjuvants to enhance vaccine responses has generated interest in heat-shock proteins (HSPs).[64] Various forms of cellular stress, such as hypoxia, pharmacologic agents, or heat, can cause increased synthesis of HSPs, which act as intracellular chaperones to bind, assemble, and disaggregate proteins.[65] When released extracellularly, HSPs are potent immune stimulators, as they enhance antigen processing and presentation.[66] Although clinical trials using HSPs as adjuvants in sarcoma have yet to be realized, preclinical literature to support this approach is growing. The use of HSPs derived from tumors enhances immune responses to MCA-induced sarcomas and protects against tumor establishment in mouse models.[45] HSPs can serve as immune stimulators or as potential targets, as their expression may be unique to certain tumor types. In a series of in vitro experiments, HSP72 was predominantly found in tumor cells in culture, specifically Ewing sarcoma and osteosarcoma cells, in comparison with normal cells from healthy human volunteers.[67] After a nonlethal heat stress at 41.8°C and a recovery period at 37°C, HSP72 was found in these cell lines to be localized to the cell membrane rather than within the cells. The heat-shock–inducible tumor-specific HSP72 cell-surface expression was associated with an increased sensitivity to lysis mediated by NK cells stimulated by IL-2, and was not dependent on tumor cell expression of MHC I.[68,69] In general, it is thought that because particular HSP expression is limited to tumor cells in vitro, the ability to induce an antitumor immune response resulting in cell death in vivo may be a possibility.

Hyperthermia has shown promise in enhancing the effects of chemotherapy and radiation therapy in the clinical treatment of sarcomas, and is being explored as an adjuvant to immunotherapies.[70,71] The combination of immunotherapy and hyperthermia was investigated in a preclinical model of MCA 105 sarcomas. Mice were treated with whole-body hyperthermia alone, immunotherapy with tumor-sensitized lymphocytes, or whole-body hyperthermia and immunotherapy. A significant reduction in growth of both primary extremity sarcomas and pulmonary metastases was noted.[72,73] The use of hyperthermia as an adjunct to immunotherapy for human sarcomas has yet to be fully characterized, but it may ultimately prove to be a nontoxic and effective adjuvant.

Adoptive Immunotherapy

Adoptive immunotherapy, involving the transfer of preconditioned immune reactive cells to a tumor-bearing patient, has been extensively studied.[74] Preclinical data have demonstrated that the transfer of tumor-infiltrating lymphocytes (TIL) expanded with IL-2 into mice with pulmonary or hepatic metastases from MCA 105 sarcoma resulted in a 50% cure rate.[75] A caveat to the transfer of TILs from human tumors, including sarcoma, is that although the culture of TILs could be established, the T lymphocytes are phenotypically heterogeneous and do not remain constant during prolonged time in culture.[76] Considering a different approach in the pediatric population, NK cells were collected from peripheral blood of healthy adult patients and sensitized with Ewing sarcoma, rhabdomyosarcoma, neuroblastoma, and osteosarcoma cell lines. Ewing sarcoma cells appeared to be the most sensitive to the cytotoxicity of expanded activated NK cells.[77]

These findings were recently extended to a clinical application of adoptive immunotherapy in patients with synovial cell sarcoma. Autologous T cells were transduced with T-cell receptors capable of recognizing NY-ESO-1, a cancer/testis antigen (CTA) that is overexpressed in the majority of synovial cell sarcomas.[75] In a clinical trial using these genetically engineered T cells combined with IL-2, two-thirds of patients with synovial cell sarcoma had objective clinical responses. One patient showed a partial response that was durable for 18 months. This study showed that sarcomas might be susceptible to adoptive immunotherapy protocols and that a targeted approach could result in profound clinical responses.

Role of Other Immune-Associated Molecules

Further insight into T-cell activation and function involves an understanding of the role of cytotoxic T-lymphocyte antigen 4 (CTLA-4). Preclinical studies have shown that T cells are inhibited by CTLA-4, which is undetectable on freshly isolated T cells but is detected in significant amounts 48 hours after T-cell stimulation. As a likely feedback loop mechanism, CTLA-4 strongly inhibits T-cell proliferation as well as IL-2 secretion by T cells.[78] The theory that the combination of a vaccine with anti–CTLA-4 antibody would enhance the T-cell response to the vaccine was tested in two mouse models: a meth A sarcoma cell line and a primary prostate tumor cell line.[79,80] Results of these studies and others indicate augmentation of the immune response when anti–CTLA-4 antibody is added at the time of immunotherapy.[81] Clinical trials involving the anti–CTLA-4 antibody, ipilimumab (Yervoy; Bristol-Myers Squibb, New York, NY), have been completed in melanoma, in which an objective response rate of 15% has been reported to the antibody alone.[82] Concomitant administration of ipilimumab with sarcoma vaccines has not yet been studied in clinical trials, but results from melanoma studies suggest this may be relevant.

FUTURE DIRECTIONS

Studies in immunotherapy for sarcoma have been challenged by the heterogeneous nature of this group of tumors. The identification of sarcoma TAAs is central to this, and the search has involved investigation of several possibilities (**Table 2**). CTAs are antigens mostly limited to germline cells and cancer cells. CTAs are frequently expressed in tumors of some histologic types (eg, NY-ESO-1 in synovial cell sarcomas), but infrequently in others. A study of CTA expression in sarcoma tumors and cell lines found that CTAs were expressed in clusters, with multiple CTAs being simultaneously present in the same tumor.[83] As the immune response to these

Table 2
Sarcoma tumor-associated antigens (TAA)

	TAA	Comment
Protein products	SYT-SSX fusion protein	Synovial sarcoma
	p53, erbB2, MDM2, c-KIT	Sarcoma associated with Li Fraumeni syndrome
Viral antigens	HHV8	Kaposi sarcoma
Chromosomal translocations	t(X:18)(p11;q11) t(11;22)(q24;q12)	Synovial sarcoma Ewing sarcoma
Cancer testis antigens	NY-ESO1	Synovial sarcoma

CTAs selectively targets cancer cells, these molecules are good candidates for the development of vaccine or adoptive immunotherapy strategies.

Genetic abnormalities are known to be an important factor in the development of sarcomas. Overexpressed protein products such as p53, erbB2, MDM2, and c-KIT are thought to be possible targets for the development of immunotherapies.[84] In addition, sarcomas often have specific chromosomal translocations resulting in production of fusion proteins, for example the characteristic t(X;18)(p11;q11) translocation of synovial sarcoma. These fusion proteins are specific to each particular sarcoma, making them ideal targets for immunotherapy, particularly in pediatric sarcomas.[85]

SUMMARY

Based on initial observations, the effect of the host immune system on STS has become increasingly clear. The immune system plays a critical role in both the development and growth of sarcomas. Translating preclinical findings for the treatment of sarcomas in humans has begun, with varying degrees of success. Future improvements in immunotherapy strategies for sarcoma will involve the use of novel adjuvants or costimulatory molecules currently under development. The success of future immunotherapies for sarcoma is dependent on further discovery of TAAs that will allow for targeted immunotherapies in this heterogeneous group of tumors.

REFERENCES

1. Jemal A, Bray F, Center MM, et al. Global cancer statistics. CA Cancer J Clin 2011;61:69–90.
2. Gibault L, Perot G, Chibon F, et al. New insights in sarcoma oncogenesis: a comprehensive analysis of a large series of 160 soft tissue sarcomas with complex genomics. J Pathol 2011;223:64–71.
3. Randall RL, Bruckner JD, Papenhausen MD, et al. Errors in diagnosis and margin determination of soft-tissue sarcomas initially treated at non-tertiary centers. Orthopedics 2004;27(2):209–12.
4. McCarthy EF. The toxins of William B. Coley and the treatment of bone and soft-tissue sarcomas. Iowa Orthop J 2006;26:154–8.
5. Coley WB. The treatment of malignant tumors by repeated inoculations of Erysipelas: with a report of ten original cases. Am J Med Sci 1893;10:487–511.
6. Coley WB. Contribution to the knowledge of sarcoma. Ann Surg 1891;14:199–220.
7. The failure of the erysipelas toxins [editorial]. JAMA 1894;24:919.
8. Coley-Nauts H, McLaren JR. Coley toxins—the first century. Adv Exp Med Biol 1990;267:483–500.
9. Johnston B, Novales ET. Clinical effects of Coley's toxin: a seven year study. Cancer Chemother Rep 1962;21:43–68.
10. Carswell EA, Old LJ, Kassel RL, et al. An endotoxin-induced serum factor that causes necrosis of tumors. Proc Natl Acad Sci U S A 1975;72(9):3666–70.
11. Tsung K, Norton JA. Lessons from Coley's toxin. Surg Oncol 2006;15(1):25–8.
12. Burnet FM. Cancer—a biological approach. Br Med J 1957;1:841–7.
13. Burnet FM. Immunological factors in the process of carcinogenesis. Br Med Bull 1964;20:154–8.
14. Burnet FM. The concept of immunological surveillance. Prog Exp Tumor Res 1970;13:1–127.
15. Dunn GP, Bruce AT, Ikeda H, et al. Cancer immunoediting: from immunosurveillance to tumor escape. Nat Immunol 2002;3(11):991–8.

16. Koebel CM, Vermi W, Swann JB, et al. Adaptive immunity maintains occult cancer in an equilibrium state. Nature 2007;450(7171):903–7.
17. Swann JB, Vesely MD, Silva A, et al. Demonstration of inflammation-induced cancer and cancer immunoediting during primary tumorigenesis. Proc Natl Acad Sci U S A 2008;105(2):652–8.
18. Zhang L, Conejo-Garcia JR, Katsaros D, et al. Intratumoral T cells, recurrence, and survival in epithelial ovarian cells. N Engl J Med 2003;348(3):203–13.
19. Berghuis D, Santos SJ, Baelde HJ, et al. Pro-inflammatory chemokine-chemokine receptor interactions within the Ewing sarcoma microenvironment determine CD8(+) T-lymphocyte infiltration and affect tumour progression. J Pathol 2011; 223(3):347–57.
20. Brinkrolf P, Landmeier S, Altvater B, et al. A high proportion of bone marrow T cells with regulatory phenotype (CD4+CD25^{hi}FoxP3+) in Ewing sarcoma patients is associated with metastatic disease. Int J Cancer 2009;125(4): 879–86.
21. Dalen BP, Geijer M, Kvist H, et al. Clinical and imaging observations of desmoid tumors left without treatment. Acta Orthoped 2006;77(6):932–7.
22. Nakayama T, Tsuboyama T, Toguchida J, et al. Natural course of desmoid-type fibromatosis. J Orthop Sci 2008;13(1):51–5.
23. Matsuo T, Shimose S, Kubo T, et al. Extraskeletal osteosarcoma with partial spontaneous regression. Anticancer Res 2009;29:5197–202.
24. Noria S, David A, Kandel R, et al. Residual disease following unplanned excision of a soft-tissue sarcoma of an extremity. J Bone Joint Surg 1996;78(5):650–5.
25. Lewis JJ, Leung D, Espat J, et al. Effect of reresection in extremity soft tissue sarcoma. Ann Surg 2000;5:655–63.
26. Tsukahara T, Kawaguchi S, Torigoe T, et al. Prognostic significance of HLA class I expression in osteosarcoma defined by anti-pan HLA class I monoclonal antibody, EMR8-5. Cancer Sci 2006;97(12):1374–80.
27. Mitchell MS. Immunology of sarcomas. Clin Orthop Rel Res 1980;153:26–30.
28. Morton DL, Malmgren RA. Human osteosarcomas: immunologic evidence suggesting an associated infectious agent. Science 1968;162(3859):1279–81.
29. Morton DL, Malmgren RA, Hall WT, et al. Immunologic and virus studies with human sarcomas. Surgery 1969;66(1):152–61.
30. Wood WC, Morton DL. Host immune response to a common cell-surface antigen in human sarcomas: detection by cytotoxicity tests. N Engl J Med 1971;284(11):569–72.
31. Gupta RK, Morton DL. Detection of cancer-associated antigen(s) in urine of sarcoma patients. J Surg Oncol 1979;11(1):65–74.
32. Mesri EA, Cesarman E, Boshoff C. Kaposi's sarcoma and its associated herpesvirus. Nat Rev Cancer 2010;10:707–19.
33. Ledergerber B, Telenti A, Egger M. Risk of HIV related Kaposi's sarcoma and non-Hodgkin's lymphoma with potent antiretroviral therapy: prospective cohort study. Swiss HIV Cohort Study. Br Med J 1999;319:23–4.
34. Wilkinson J, Cope A, Gill J, et al. Identification of Kaposi's sarcoma-associated herpesvirus (KSHV)-specific cytotoxic T-lymphocyte epitopes and evaluation of reconstitution of KSHV-specific responses in human immunodeficiency virus type 1-infected patients receiving highly active antiretroviral therapy. J Virol 2002;76(6):2634–40.
35. Gill J, Bourboulia D, Wilkinson J, et al. Prospective study of the effects of antiretroviral therapy on Kaposi sarcoma-associated herpesvirus infection in patients with and without Kaposi sarcoma. J Acquir Immune Defic Syndr 2002;31: 384–90.

36. DeLeo AB, Jay G, Appella E, et al. Detection of a transformation-related antigen in chemically induced sarcomas and other transformed cells of the mouse. Proc Natl Acad Sci U S A 1979;76(5):2420–4.

37. North RJ, Bursuker I. Generation and decay of the immune response to a progressive fibrosarcoma. J Exp Med 1984;159:1295–311.

38. Shu S, Rosenberg SA. Adoptive immunotherapy of newly induced murine sarcomas. Cancer Res 1985;45:1657–62.

39. Chou T, Chang AE, Shu S. Generation of therapeutic T lymphocytes from tumor-bearing mice by in vitro sensitization: culture requirements and characterization of immunologic specificity. J Immunol 1988;140(7):2453–61.

40. Shu S, Rosenberg SA. Adoptive immunotherapy of a newly induced sarcoma: immunologic characteristics of effector cells. J Immunol 1985;135(4):2895–903.

41. Chou T, Bertera S, Chang AE, et al. Adoptive immunotherapy of microscopic and advanced visceral metastases with in vitro sensitized lymphoid cells from mice bearing progressive tumors. J Immunol 1988;141(5):1775–81.

42. Basse P, Herberman RB, Nannmark U, et al. Accumulation of adoptively transferred adherent, lymphokine-activated killer cells in murine metastases. J Exp Med 1991;174(2):479–88.

43. Shiloni E, Lafreniere R, Mule JJ, et al. Effect of immunotherapy with allogeneic lymphokine-activated killer cells and recombinant interleukin 2 on established pulmonary and hepatic metastases in mice. Cancer Res 1986;46(11): 5633–40.

44. Sabel MS, Arora A, Su G, et al. Synergistic effect of intratumoral IL-12 and TNF-alpha microspheres: systemic antitumor immunity is mediated by both CD8+ CTL and NK cells. Surgery 2007;142(5):749–60.

45. Guo QY, Yuan M, Peng J, et al. Antitumor activity of mixed heat shock protein/peptide vaccine and cyclophosphamide plus interleukin-12 in mice sarcoma. J Exp Clin Cancer Res 2011;30(1):24–30.

46. Tevz G, Kranjc S, Cemazar M, et al. Controlled systemic release of interleukin-12 after gene electrotransfer to muscle for cancer gene therapy alone or in combination with ionizing radiation in murine sarcomas. J Gene Med 2009;11(12): 1125–37.

47. Kennel SJ, Lankford T, Flynn KM. Therapy of a murine sarcoma using syngeneic monoclonal antibody. Cancer Res 1983;43:2843–8.

48. Kennel SJ, Lankford PK, Flynn KM, et al. Factors affecting passive monoclonal antibody therapy of Moloney sarcoma in BALB/c mice. Cancer Res 1985;45: 3782–9.

49. Rosenberg SA, Yang JC, Restifo NP. Cancer immunotherapy: moving beyond current vaccines. Nature Med 2004;10(9):909–15.

50. Marcove RC, Mike V, Huvos AG, et al. Vaccine trials for osteogenic sarcoma: a preliminary report. CA Cancer J Clin 1973;23(2):74–80.

51. Marcove RC, Southam CM, Levin A, et al. A clinical trial of autogenous vaccine in osteogenic sarcoma in patients under the age of twenty-five. Surg Forum 1971; 22:434–5.

52. Dillman RO, Wiemann M, Nayak SK, et al. Interferon-gamma or granulocyte-macrophage colony-stimulating factor administered as adjuvants with a vaccine of irradiated autologous tumor cells from short-term cell line cultures: a randomized phase 2 trial of the cancer biotherapy research group. J Immunother 2003; 26(4):367–73.

53. Morgan J, Spendlove I, Durrant LG. The role of CD55 in protecting the tumour environment from complement attack. Tissue Antigens 2002;60(3):213–23.

54. Pritchard-Jones K, Spendlove I, Wilton C, et al. Douglas, and. Immune response to the 105AD7 human anti-idiotypic vaccine after intensive chemotherapy, for osteosarcoma. Br J Cancer 2005;92:1358–65.

55. Melief CJ. Cancer immunotherapy by dendritic cells. Immunity 2008;29:372–83.

56. Banchereau J, Steinman RM. Dendritic cells and the control of immunity. Nature 1998;392:245–52.

57. Geiger J, Hutchinson R, Hohenkirk L, et al. Treatment of solid tumors in children with tumor-lysate-pulsed dendritic cells. Lancet 2000;356:1163–5.

58. Matsuzaki A, Suminoe A, Hattori H, et al. Immunotherapy with autologous dendritic cells and tumor-specific synthetic peptides for synovial sarcoma. J Pediatr Hematol Oncol 2002;24(3):220–3.

59. Mackall CL, Rhee EH, Read EJ, et al. A pilot study of consolidative immuno-therapy in patients with high-risk pediatric sarcomas. Clin Cancer Res 2008; 14(15):4850–8.

60. Maki RG. Future directions for immunotherapeutic intervention against sarcomas. Curr Opin Oncol 2006;18:363–8.

61. Dranoff G, Jaffee E, Lazenby A, et al. Vaccination with irradiated tumor cells en-gineered to secrete murine granulocyte-macrophage colony-stimulating factor stimulates potent, specific, and long-lasting anti-tumor immunity. Proc Natl Acad Sci U S A 1993;90:3539–43.

62. Mahvi DM, Shi FS, Yang NS, et al. Immunization by particle-mediated transfer of the granulocyte-macrophage colony stimulating factor gene into autologous tumor cells in melanoma or sarcoma patients: report of a phase I/IB study. Hum Gene Ther 2002;13:1711–21.

63. Dagher R, Long LM, Read EJ, et al. Pilot trial of tumor-specific peptide vaccina-tion and continuous infusion interleukin-2 in patients with recurrent Ewing sarcoma and alveolar rhabdomyosarcoma: an inter-interinstitute NIH study. Med Pediatr Oncol 2002;38:158–64.

64. Lindquist S. The heat shock response. Annu Rev Biochem 1986;55:1151–91.

65. Chirico WJ, Waters MG, Blobel G. 70K heat shock related proteins stimulate protein translocation into microsomes. Nature 1988;332:805–10.

66. Vanbuskirk A, Crump BL, Margoliash E, et al. A peptide binding protein having a role in antigen presentation is a member of the HSP70 heat shock family. J Exp Med 1989;170:1799–809.

67. Multhoff G, Botzler C, Wiesnet M, et al. A stress-inducible 72-kDa heat shock protein (HSP 72) is expressed on the surface of human tumor cells, but not on normal cells. Int J Cancer 1995;61:272–9.

68. Multhoff G, Botzler C, Wiesnet M, et al. CD3- large granular lymphocytes recog-nize a heat-inducible immunogenic determinant associated with the 72-kD heat shock protein on human sarcoma cells. Blood 1995;86(4):1374–82.

69. Multhoff G. Heat shock protein 72 (HSP72), a hyperthermia inducible immuno-genic determinant on leukemic K562 and Ewing's sarcoma cells. Int J Hyper-thermia 1997;13(1):39–48.

70. Issels RD, Lindner LH, Verweij J, et al. European Organization for Research and Treatment of Cancer Soft Tissue and Bone Sarcoma Group (EORTC-STBSG): Euro-pean Society for Hyperthermic Oncology (ESHO). Neo-adjuvant chemotherapy alone or with regional hyperthermia for localized high-risk soft tissue sarcoma: a randomized phase 3 multicenter study. Lancet Oncol 2010;11(6):561–70.

71. Otsuka T, Yonezawa M, Kamiyama F, et al. Results of surgery and radio-hyperthermo-chemotherapy for patients with soft tissue sarcoma. Int J Clin Oncol 2001;6(5):253–8.

72. Geehan DM, Fabian DF, Lefor AT. Immunotherapy and whole body hyperthermia as combined modality treatment of a subcutaneous murine sarcoma. J Surg Oncol 1993;53:180–3.
73. Strauch ED, Fabian DF, Turner J, et al. Combined hyperthermia and immunotherapy treatment of multiple pulmonary metastases in mice. Surg Oncol 1994; 3:45–52.
74. Gattinoni L, Powell DJ, Rosenberg SA, et al. Adoptive immunotherapy for cancer: building on success. Nature Immunol 2006;6:383–93.
75. Rosenberg SA, Spiess P, Lafreniere R. A new approach to the adoptive immunotherapy of cancer with tumor-infiltrating lymphocytes. Science 1986;233: 1318–21.
76. Schiltz PM, Beutel LD, Nayak SK, et al. Characterization of tumor-infiltrating lymphocytes derived from human tumors for use as adoptive immunotherapy of cancer. J Immunother 1997;20(5):377–86.
77. Cho D, Shook DR, Shimasaki N, et al. Cytotoxicity of activated natural killer cells against pediatric solid tumors. Clin Cancer Res 2010;16:3901–9.
78. Krummel MF, Allison JP. CD28 and CTLA-4 have opposing effects on the response of T cells to stimulation. J Exp Med 1995;182:459–65.
79. Daftarian P, Song GY, Ali S, et al. Two distinct pathways of immuno-modulation improve potency of p53 immunization in rejecting established tumors. Cancer Res 2004;64:5407–14.
80. Hurwitz AA, Foster BA, Kwon ED, et al. Combination immunotherapy of primary prostate cancer in a transgenic mouse model using CTLA-4 blockade. Cancer Res 2000;60:2444–8.
81. Espenschied J, Lamont J, Longmate J, et al. CTLA-4 blockade enhances the therapeutic effect of an attenuated poxvirus vaccine targeting p53 in an established murine tumor model. J Immunol 2003;170:3401–7.
82. Hodi FS, O'Day SJ, McDermott DF, et al. Improved survival with ipilimumab in patients with metastatic melanoma. N Engl J Med 2010;363(8):711–23.
83. Ayyoub M, Taub RN, Keohan ML, et al. The frequent expression of cancer/testis antigens provides opportunities for immunotherapeutic targeting of sarcoma. Cancer Immun 2004;4:7–14.
84. Todd R, Lunec J. Molecular pathology and potential therapeutic targets in soft-tissue sarcoma. Expert Rev Anticancer Ther 2008;8(6):939–48.
85. Goletz T, Mackall CL, Berzofsky JA, et al. Molecular alterations in pediatric sarcomas: potential targets for immunotherapy. Sarcoma 1998;2:77–87.

Index

Note: Page numbers of article titles are in **boldface** type.

A

Ablative therapy, nonsurgical, for pulmonary metastases of soft tissue sarcoma, 279–280
Adipocytic tumors, atypical lipomatous tumor *vs.* well-differentiated liposarcoma, **333–340**
Adjuvant therapy, after pulmonary metastasectomy, 277–279
    chemotherapy, 277–279
    radiation, 277
  chemotherapy for soft tissue sarcomas, **243–253**
    histology-specific trials of, 249–251
      bone sarcoma, 250–251
      gastrointestinal stromal tumors, 251
      leiomyosarcoma, 250
      liposarcoma, 250
      synovial sarcoma, 249–250
    neoadjuvant, 248–249
    systemic, 244–248
  chemotherapy plus radiation for extremity and truncal soft tissue sarcomas, 229
  for primary resectable gastrointestinal stromal tumors, 305–306
  preoperative *vs.* postoperative radiation for extremity soft tissue sarcomas, 218–219
  radiation for retroperitoneal sarcoma, 325–327
Adjuvants, use in vaccines sarcomas, clinical data for, 348–349
Adoptive immunotherapy, for sarcomas, clinical data for, 349–350
Adriamycin, for adjuvant chemotherapy of soft tissue sarcomas, 244–245
    ifosfamide and, 245–248
    meta-analysis of trials of, 248
Amputation, for soft tissue sarcomas of extremities, 210
Atypical lipomatous tumor, *vs.* well-differentiated liposarcomas, **333–340**

B

Biopsy, diagnostic, for soft tissue sarcomas, 191
Bone sarcomas, histology-specific adjuvant chemotherapy trials for, 250–251
Brachytherapy, for extremity and truncal soft tissue sarcomas, 218–220
  for soft tissue sarcomas of extremities, 206–207

C

Chemotherapy, adjuvant, after pulmonary metastasectomy, 277–279
  adjuvant, for soft tissue sarcomas, **243–253**
    histology-specific trials of, 249–251
      bone sarcoma, 250–251
      gastrointestinal stromal tumors, 251
      leiomyosarcoma, 250
      liposarcoma, 250

Surg Oncol Clin N Am 21 (2012) 357–366
doi:10.1016/S1055-3207(12)00013-0
1055-3207/12/$ – see front matter © 2012 Elsevier Inc. All rights reserved.

surgonc.theclinics.com

Moving?

Make sure your subscription moves with you!

To notify us of your new address, find your **Clinics Account Number** (located on your mailing label above your name), and contact customer service at:

Email: journalscustomerservice-usa@elsevier.com

800-654-2452 (subscribers in the U.S. & Canada)
314-447-8871 (subscribers outside of the U.S. & Canada)

Fax number: 314-447-8029

Elsevier Health Sciences Division
Subscription Customer Service
3251 Riverport Lane
Maryland Heights, MO 63043

*To ensure uninterrupted delivery of your subscription, please notify us at least 4 weeks in advance of move.

Printed and bound by CPI Group (UK) Ltd, Croydon, CR0 4YY

03/10/2024

01040458-0018